PROTECT YOUR CUPCAKES

Understanding & Fighting Breast Cancer

Raquell Stuart

Protect Your Cupcakes: Understanding & Fighting Breast Cancer — Expanded Edition

Published by Blue Horizon Books • Plantation, Florida • Nassau, The Bahamas

Revived & Expanded Edition, 2026. Printed worldwide.

ISBN: 978-0-578-64869-9

Publication history: original manuscript © 2020; revived and expanded edition © 2026.

Book Categories:

- Health & Wellness / Breast Cancer Awareness
- Medical / Oncology / Patient Education
- Caribbean Studies / Public Health
- Young Adult Nonfiction / Health

Revived & Expanded Edition — 2026

 This edition preserves the original youth voice while adding new chapters, updated illustrations, Bahamian and Caribbean context, and a source review updated through September 2026.

Disclaimer: This book is for education and awareness only and is not medical advice. Screening, genetic testing, diagnosis, and treatment decisions depend on age, personal risk, family history, country, and clinical circumstances. Guidance changes over time. Readers should discuss personal health concerns with a qualified healthcare professional.

Dedication

For every woman in my family, and in every family,
who has ever heard the word "cancer"
and chosen to keep going.

For my aunt Lorna, whose courage is half the reason this book exists.

For my grandfather, Clyde Ifill, whose memory keeps me studying.

And for my mom and dad, who never let me stop writing it.

— R. S.

A Note from Raquell

(Author's Note)

This book didn't start in a bedroom with a notebook. It started on a stage at Queens College.

When I was named Student of the Year, part of the honour was choosing a platform — a cause I cared about enough to fundraise for, speak about, and build a campaign around. With the help of my parents and Mrs. Sylvia Beneby, I chose breast cancer. I chose it because the stories were everywhere. So many Bahamian women were being diagnosed, so many families were being shaken, and yet nobody in my class could clearly explain what breast cancer actually was. That didn't feel right.

That platform gave me a voice. It allowed me to raise money for women affected by breast cancer and to partner with the Cancer Society of The Bahamas to support their work and spread awareness across the country. It also pushed me further than I ever imagined — to First Runner-Up for National Student of the Year, out of every high school in The Bahamas. Getting there took hours of speeches, fundraisers, rehearsals, and research, and it changed what I believed one young person could do.

Protect Your Cupcakes started during that same year. I was thirteen, and I kept thinking: talking about breast cancer isn't enough. People need something they can read. Something written by someone their age. Something that explains this disease in a way that doesn't scare you out of paying attention. I chose the name because "cupcakes" is what a lot of girls my age jokingly call their breasts — sweet, ours, and worth protecting.

This book also became personal. A few years after I wrote the first draft, my aunt faced a serious diagnosis and underwent major surgery, including a hysterectomy. Our family walked every step with her — the scans, the surgery, the waiting, the recovery. It changed everything. I was not writing about other people's families anymore. I was writing about mine.

I also carry the memory of my grandfather, Clyde Ifill, who passed away from pancreatic cancer. Losing him left a mark on my life and strengthened my desire to become an oncologist — someone who doesn't just study cancer, but stands with people through it.

A lot has changed since the grade 8 version of me wrote the first draft. The facts have been updated. I've grown. But the reason this book exists hasn't changed: girls, women, moms, aunts, grandmas, sisters — and even boys and men — deserve to understand breast cancer and know what we can do about it.

When my dad and I sat down to revive this book in 2026, we made a decision together: we would keep the voice of the thirteen-year-old who started it. That voice is honest, curious, sometimes funny, and never pretends to be a doctor. I am not a doctor — not yet. I am a student who did the work to learn. I checked everything carefully, with guidance from my mom, who works in medicine, and from trusted research sources. If something here worries you, please talk to a parent or a doctor. And if something here helps you, pass it on.

Thank you for letting me be a part of your story. I hope this book becomes a part of it.

Raquell Stuart

WHERE IT ALL BEGAN

Raquell's original Bahamas breast-cancer awareness campaign

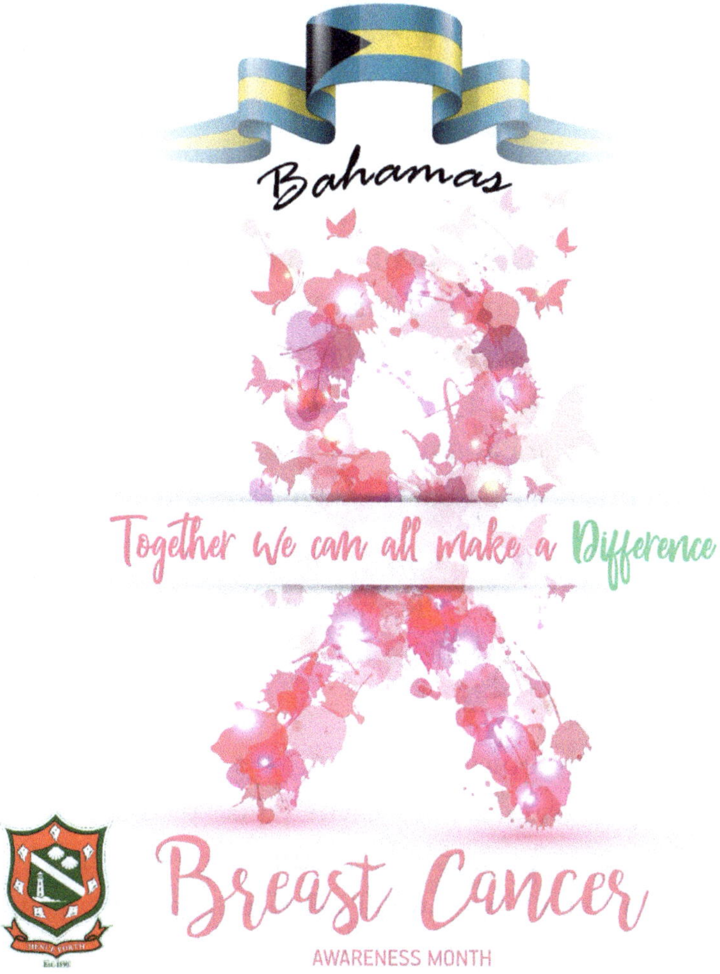

Original Student of the Year breast-cancer awareness banner used during Raquell's Queen's College campaign.

Before this was a book, breast-cancer awareness was my cause. At thirteen, I used this banner during my Student of the Year campaign at Queen's College to help people learn, talk, fundraise, and take action. The message — "Together we can all make a difference" — still belongs in this book. The campaign became the first edition in 2020 and this revived edition in 2026.

A Note from Mom & Dad

The first draft of this book sat in a folder on our computer for almost six years. Every so often, we would open it, read a page, and close it again, thinking: someday.

That someday is now.

Our daughter, Raquell, began Protect Your Cupcakes during her Student of the Year journey at Queens College. She not only represented her school but went on to become First Runner-Up for National Student of the Year across The Bahamas. Her platform was breast cancer, and she approached it with purpose — raising funds, speaking to audiences, partnering with the Cancer Society of The Bahamas, and still finding the discipline to begin writing this book at just thirteen years old.

That kind of commitment does not happen in isolation. We are deeply grateful to Queens College, to its leadership, and especially to Mrs. Sylvia Beneby, whose guidance and care helped shape the young woman behind these pages.

Cancer is not just a topic in this book — it is part of our family's story. Raquell's grandfather, Clyde Ifill, passed away from pancreatic cancer. His loss is something we still carry, and it played a role in shaping Raquell's desire to pursue a future in oncology — to understand the disease and stand with others through it. We also walked through the diagnosis, treatment, and recovery of Raquell's aunt, and saw how the small acts of a family — the rides, the meals, the sitting together in waiting rooms — form the real support structure that hospitals cannot provide.

We are also grateful for the role that medicine has played in this journey. As her mother works in the medical field, her guidance helped ensure that this book remained grounded in accuracy, responsibility, and care. Every statistic was double-checked. Every medical term was reviewed. Every chapter in this expanded edition has been re-sourced using current guidance from trusted institutions including the American Cancer Society, the National Cancer Institute, the Pan American Health Organization, the World Health Organization, Susan G. Komen, the National Comprehensive Cancer Network, and peer-reviewed Bahamian BRCA1 research.

We extend a sincere thank you to the Fox Foundation for its leadership in breast cancer awareness in The Bahamas, particularly through the provision of free breast exams during Breast Cancer Awareness Month. Efforts like these are not just helpful — they are life-saving.

In The Bahamas, breast cancer affects women earlier and more aggressively than in many parts of the world. Too many people still do not understand why, and too many are unaware that early detection can save lives. We hope this book changes that, one reader at a time.

This revived and expanded edition preserves Raquell's voice while strengthening the science behind it. New chapters on nutrition and lifestyle, on young people and family, and on how ordinary students can become advocates make this a book for every age group — not just the patient and her doctors.

Thank you for picking up this book. If it leads even one person to take action — to check, to ask, to learn — then it has fulfilled its purpose. And if it inspires one young person to pick up a pen or a microscope or a microphone and fight for the women in their lives, then it has done more than we ever hoped.

With love and pride,

— Mom & Dad

Acknowledgements

There is no version of this book without Queens College. It was more than a school — it was the place that taught me a student could take action on what she cares about. The Student of the Year journey, the platform, the fundraisers, the speeches, the late nights — all of it was possible because Queens College believed that students could lead. To every teacher, administrator, and staff member: thank you.

A special thank you to the Principal, Mr. Henry Knowles, and the Vice Principal, whose leadership created the kind of environment where a big idea could actually grow.

And to Mrs. Sylvia Beneby — there are not enough words. You were my coach, my mentor, and a mother to me throughout this journey. You showed up for every rehearsal, every draft, every difficult moment. You believed in me before I believed in myself. This book carries your influence on every page, and I will be grateful for you for the rest of my life.

Thank you to the Cancer Society of The Bahamas and the Sister Sister Breast Cancer Support Group for welcoming a young student into work that truly matters. The funds raised through my platform were placed in your hands — hands that have been doing this work for decades — and I am honored to have played a small part.

To my mom, thank you for answering my questions, even in the middle of everyday life, and for guiding me with patience and love. You were my first teacher.

To my aunt, thank you for trusting me with your story. Your strength is woven into this book.

To my dad, thank you for answering every question, for bringing this book back to life after six years, and for reminding me that it was time to finish what I started.

Thank you to my teachers at Queens College who showed me that meaningful work does not need to be assigned to matter. And to my science teacher — thank you for letting me bring a breast anatomy model into class and making it normal.

Thank you to the organizations and researchers whose work made this book possible, including Susan G. Komen, the American Cancer Society, the Pan American Health Organization (PAHO), the World Health Organization, the National Cancer Institute, the Breast Cancer Research Foundation, the Fox Foundation, and the research teams of Dr. Judith Hurley and Dr. Mohammad Akbari, whose landmark BRCA1 study changed what we know about Bahamian women.

Thank you to the many survivors whose memoirs, interviews, blog posts, and podcasts taught me how to listen. I cannot list you all — but your courage is everywhere in this book.

And to you, the reader — thank you for opening this book. That is where change begins.

How to Use This Book

You do not have to read this book front to back. You do not have to read all of it in one sitting. This is a book you can open, close, put down, pick back up, and write inside of.

Here are a few ways different readers might want to use it:

If you are a student (ages 11–17):

Start with the Introduction, Chapter 1 (What Is Breast Cancer?), and Chapter 5 (Breast Awareness & Early Detection). Those three pieces give you the basic map. Then flip around based on what's interesting or useful to you.

If you are a parent or older family member:

The chapters you may find most useful are Chapter 4 (Genes, Risks & BRCA), Chapter 6 (Breast Cancer in The Bahamas & the Caribbean), and Chapter 10 (Support, Family & Hope). If you are Bahamian or of Caribbean descent, Chapter 6 was written especially with you in mind.

If someone you love was just diagnosed:

I am sorry. Take a breath. Go straight to Chapter 7 (Treatments) and Chapter 10 (Support, Family & Hope). The glossary in the back will help you decode medical letters. You are not behind — you are exactly on time.

If you are a patient yourself:

You already know things this book is only trying to explain. Please use the parts that are useful to you and set aside anything that isn't. The sections on clinical trials (Chapter 7), nutrition and movement (Chapter 8), and survivorship (Chapter 10) are written with you in mind, but the rest of this book is also yours — especially the hope at the end.

If you are a teacher or youth leader:

The sidebars and infographics throughout the book are designed for classroom or group use. Any page with a colored box or diagram can be used as a discussion starter.

A few symbols you'll see:

- Colored sidebars contain the takeaway of a section in one paragraph — good for reviewing.
- Infographics and figures summarize data visually so you don't have to memorize every number.
- Quotes in italics come from survivors, researchers, or my own journal.

This is your copy. Mark it up. Write a date inside the cover. Pass it to someone who needs it. A book that sits on a shelf saves no one.

MEDICAL NOTE — USE THE LATEST GUIDANCE

This edition was rechecked against 2026 American Cancer Society material, National Cancer Institute resources, the 2024 USPSTF screening recommendation, PAHO/WHO reporting, and peer-reviewed Bahamian BRCA research. Different organizations may recommend different screening schedules. Personal risk always matters.

Table of CONTENTS

A Note from Raquell v
A Note from Mom & Dad ix
Acknowledgements xi
How to Use This Book xiii
Why I Wrote This Book 1
What Is Breast Cancer? 5
Breasts 101 7
What "cancer" actually means 8
How it spreads 10
Men get breast cancer too 11
Myths vs. facts 12
Types of Breast Cancer 14
Non-invasive: still in its lane 16
Invasive: out of its lane 17
Rare types you should still know 17
The three receptors doctors test for 19
Stages & Warning Signs 21
The TNM system 22
The stages, in plain English 23
Warning signs — know what to look for 25
When to call the doctor — a flowchart 26
Genes, Risks & BRCA 29
Meet BRCA1 and BRCA2 30
How much higher is the risk? 32
Other genes that matter 32
Reading a family pedigree 33
Who should think about getting tested? 35
Other things that change the risk 36
Breast Awareness & Early Detection 38
Know your normal (breast awareness) 39
If you find something 42
Clinical exams 42

Mammograms — the gold standard ... 43
MRI, ultrasound, and other screening tools ... 45
Screening timeline at a glance ... 45
The Caribbean Breast Cancer Story: The Bahamas & Beyond ... 47
A number I couldn't stop thinking about ... 48
Why the whole Caribbean is at higher risk ... 50
A closer look by country ... 50
Why are the numbers worse here? ... 51
What we can actually do ... 52
Treatments & Integrative Care ... 55
The treatment journey, step by step ... 57
Surgery ... 58
Radiation ... 59
Chemotherapy ... 60
Hormone therapy ... 61
Targeted therapy ... 61
Immunotherapy ... 62
Clinical trials ... 62
Integrative and complementary care ... 62
Nutrition, Movement & Everyday Life ... 65
Eating to protect your cupcakes ... 66
Move your body ... 69
Sleep ... 70
Stress and mental health ... 71
Things to avoid ... 71
When Cancer Comes Home ... 72
You are allowed to ask questions ... 73
You are not the cause and not the cure ... 74
Things that might help your parent or relative ... 74
Take care of yourself, too ... 75
Body image and feeling weird about your own body ... 75
When the news is hard ... 76
A few words for boys ... 76
Support, Family & Hope ... 78
What survivors say they actually need ... 80
How to talk to someone who has been diagnosed ... 81
Caregiver burnout is real ... 81
Faith, prayer, and finding meaning ... 82

Survivorship: life after treatment 83
Living with metastatic (Stage IV) breast cancer 83
Hope is a discipline 84
How You Can Help 85
If you are a student 86
If you are an adult 87
If you are a teacher or school leader 87
If you are a community leader, business owner, or church 88
Advocacy in The Bahamas and the Caribbean 88
A challenge 89
Conclusion: Protect Your Cupcakes 90
What this book has been about 91
What I hope you walk away with 92
A final word 92
Glossary 94
Resources & Hotlines 100
If you are struggling emotionally 102
Quick Reference — Take This With You 103
Works Cited 107
About the Author 109

Why I Wrote This Book

In grade 8, I did a health class project on diseases. Most of my classmates picked things like the flu or diabetes. I picked breast cancer.

I don't fully remember why. Part of it was that every October, everything turned pink. I saw pink ribbons on cereal boxes, on football cleats, on the sides of taxis. My mom bought pink pens from her clinic because part of the money went to research. Everywhere I looked, there were reminders that breast cancer mattered — but no one around me could really explain why. I wanted to understand what all the pink actually stood for.

When I started reading, I was shocked. Breast cancer is the most common cancer in women worldwide. In the United States, the average lifetime risk is about 1 in 8. For 2026, the American Cancer Society estimates about 321,910 new invasive breast-cancer cases and about 42,140 deaths among women. Where I live, the story has its own urgency: in April 2026, PAHO/WHO reported that nearly half of women diagnosed with breast cancer in The Bahamas are under age 50 and almost half present at an advanced stage.

But here is the part that changed everything for me: finding breast cancer before it has spread is strongly linked with better outcomes. Current U.S. SEER data reported by the American Cancer Society show a 5-year relative survival rate greater than 99% for localized invasive breast cancer, 87% for regional disease, and about 32% for distant disease. Those are population averages, not predictions for any one person, but the gap shows why timely evaluation, screening when appropriate, and access to effective treatment matter.

That is why this book exists.

I realized that a lot of people, especially young people, don't learn about breast cancer until they have to — until someone in their family is diagnosed, or until they are older and suddenly expected to understand everything at once. By then, it can feel overwhelming and scary. I wanted to change that. I wanted to create something that introduces this topic early, in a way that is clear, honest, and not intimidating.

This book is for girls my age — the ones who are just starting to understand their bodies. It is for their moms, sisters, aunts, and grandmas. It is for families. And it is also for the boys and men who love them, because awareness is not just a "women's issue." It is a human issue.

I also wrote this book because I didn't see many resources that sounded like me. When I was researching, a lot of the information felt distant — full of medical terms that were hard to follow and explanations that didn't feel personal. I wanted something different. I wanted something that felt like a conversation, not a lecture. Something that breaks things down simply, without taking away how serious it is.

At thirteen, I didn't have all the answers. I still don't. But I had questions, and I was willing to find answers. That is where this book started — not from expertise, but from curiosity and care.

As I kept learning, I also began to understand something bigger: knowledge is not just information. It is power. Knowing what to look for, knowing your family history, knowing when to ask questions — those things can change outcomes. They can save lives.

If you are nervous reading this, I understand. I was too. But I've learned that knowing something scary doesn't make it worse — it makes you stronger, because now you can do something about it.

This book is not meant to overwhelm you. It is meant to prepare you. It is meant to help you:

- **understand what breast cancer actually is**
- **recognize early warning signs**
- **feel confident asking questions**
- **and take simple steps to protect yourself and the people you love.**

You don't have to remember everything in one sitting. You don't have to become an expert overnight. Even learning one thing — one sign, one fact, one habit — is a step forward.

Because the truth is, small actions matter.

A conversation with your mom about family history matters.

Paying attention to your body matters.

Going for a check-up matters.

Those small moments add up, and they can make a difference.

So as you read this, take your time. Ask questions. Talk about what you learn. Share it with someone else.

Because awareness doesn't stop with you — it spreads.

And that is how we close the gap.

So grab a pink pen, find a comfortable spot, and let's protect our cupcakes.

CHAPTER ONE.

What Is Breast Cancer?

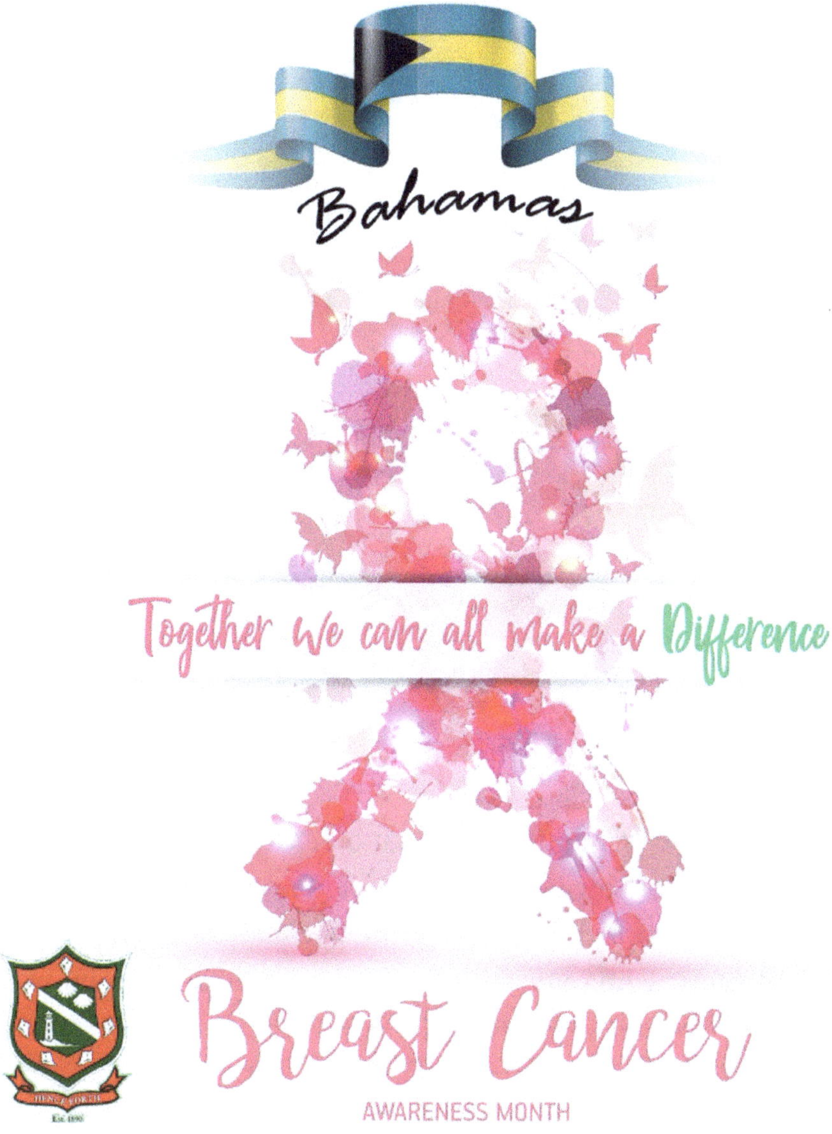

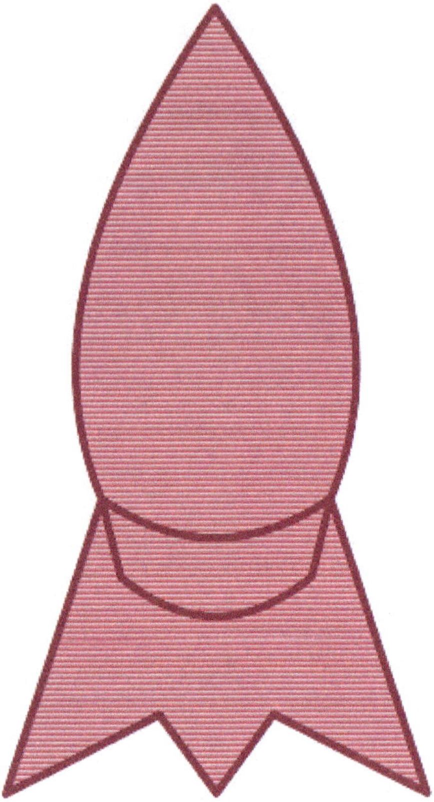

Before we can talk about breast cancer, we have to talk about breasts. That feels awkward for about ten seconds and then it stops feeling awkward, which is good, because every woman has them and every woman deserves to understand her own body.

CUPCAKE CHECK — CHAPTER 1

Breast cancer begins when breast cells grow out of control.
Most breast changes are not cancer, but new changes deserve attention.
Anyone with breast tissue can develop breast cancer.

Breasts 101

Breasts are made up of three main things: lobules, ducts, and fatty tissue. Lobules are little clusters that make milk after a baby is born. Ducts are thin tubes that carry that milk from the lobules to the nipple. Fatty tissue is the soft stuff that fills in between everything and gives the breast its shape.

Under and around all of that, there are also blood vessels and lymph nodes. Lymph nodes are tiny bean-shaped filters, mostly clustered under the arm, that help the body's immune system. You will hear about them a lot in this book, because whenever doctors talk about how "far" a cancer has spread, the lymph nodes are usually the first stop they check.

Breasts also contain ligaments — connective tissue called Cooper's ligaments — that hold the breast in shape. And they sit on top of a sheet of muscle called the pectoralis major. Cancer usually starts inside the breast itself — not in the muscle — but it can push into the muscle in later stages.

One thing most girls are never told: breast tissue actually extends past what you can see. It reaches up toward the collarbone, across to the middle of the chest, and into the armpit. That "tail" of tissue stretching into the armpit is why breast self-checks always include the underarm area. A lump can hide there and still be breast cancer.

Breasts also change throughout life. They swell and get tender before periods because of hormones. They grow during puberty. They get firmer and sometimes lumpier in the second half of the menstrual cycle. They change during pregnancy and breastfeeding. After menopause, much of the breast is replaced by fat, and the texture becomes softer. All of this is normal. None of it is cancer on its own.

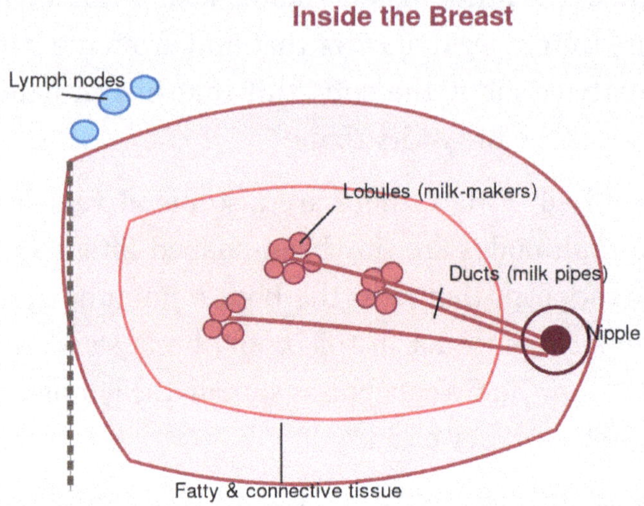

Figure 1.1 — The main parts of the breast: lobules, ducts, fat, and nearby lymph nodes.

What "cancer" actually means

Your body is made of about 37 trillion cells. Every single one of them has a built-in plan: grow, do its job, and eventually die so that new cells can take over. Cells do this all the time. When you scrape your knee and a new layer of skin grows back, that's cells following the plan perfectly.

Cancer is what happens when the plan breaks.

A normal cell has instructions inside it called DNA. Sometimes, because of something inherited (a gene you were born with), or because of damage (from things like smoking or certain chemicals), or just plain bad luck, a cell's DNA gets a mistake in it. If the mistake lands on the "stop growing" instructions, the cell starts copying itself over and over without stopping. Those copies stick together and form a lump. That lump is called a tumor.

Not all tumors are cancer. Some tumors are benign, which means they grow, but they stay in one place and don't invade anything around them. Moles and many breast cysts are benign. Cancer tumors are malignant, which means the cells break out of their lane, grow into nearby tissue, and — if you don't stop them — travel to other parts of the body.

Breast cancer is cancer that starts in breast cells. Usually, it starts in the ducts or the lobules (we will talk about the difference in Chapter 2).

Zooming in: how one cell turns into millions

This part is the part I wish someone had explained in science class. Every time a cell divides, it copies its DNA first — think of it like photocopying a very long instruction manual. That photocopy happens fast and it has to be nearly perfect. If there's a smudge (a mutation), there are backup systems in your cells — little editors called tumor suppressor genes (BRCA1 and BRCA2 are two of them) — that read over the copy and fix it.

Cancer starts when too many edits get through. Usually it takes more than one mutation. A cell needs to lose its brakes (so it grows when it shouldn't), lose its off-switch (so it doesn't die when it should), and learn to hide from the immune system (so the body doesn't kill it). That's a lot of things to go wrong — which is why cancer usually takes years to form.

That also means it has years where we could catch it. That's the good news hidden inside a scary idea.

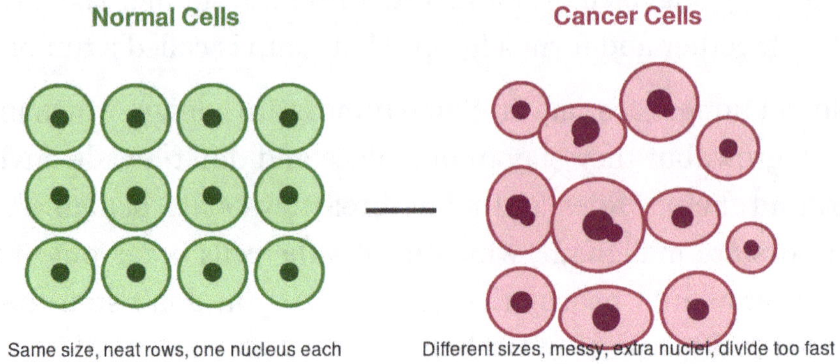

Figure 1.2 — Normal cells vs. cancer cells under a microscope.

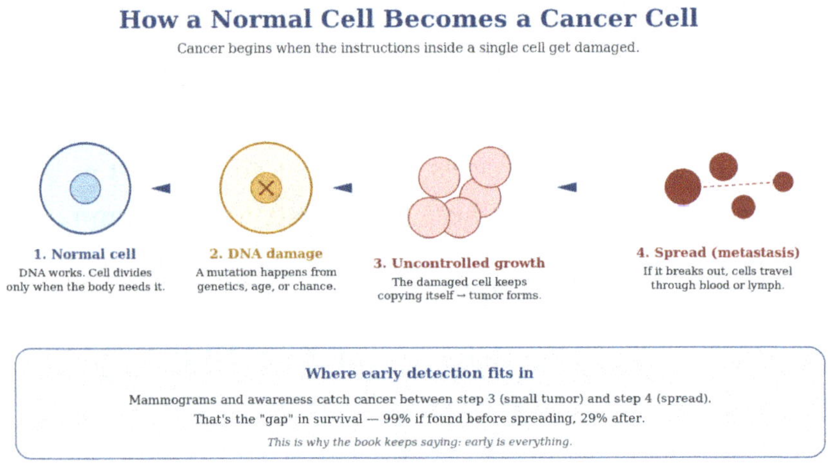

Figure 1.3 — From a normal cell to a spreading cancer: the four-step story, and where screening fits in.

How it spreads

The scariest thing about cancer is that it can travel. Doctors call this metastasis, which is a fancy word that just means "it moved."

Breast cancer spreads in two main ways:

- **Through the lymph system.** The lymph nodes under your arm are like airport security checkpoints. Sometimes cancer cells slip past and ride the lymph fluid to other places.
- **Through the bloodstream.** Blood vessels run everywhere, so once cancer cells get into them, they can end up in the lungs, liver, bones, or brain.

Breast cancer has favorite places to spread. The most common "metastatic sites" are the bones (especially the spine, ribs, and pelvis), the liver, the lungs, and the brain. When doctors say someone has "bone mets," it means the cancer that started in her breast is now also growing in her bones. The cells still behave like breast cancer cells — that's why it's treated as breast cancer, not bone cancer.

This is why, when doctors diagnose breast cancer, the first question they ask is not just "how big?" but "how far?" We will get to that when we talk about stages in Chapter 3.

Men get breast cancer too

Quick but important fact: men have breast tissue, and men can get breast cancer. It is uncommon, but real. Because people do not always expect breast cancer in men, a new lump, nipple change, or other persistent breast change should be checked rather than dismissed.

Because people don't expect it, men often find lumps later, which makes it more dangerous. The average age of diagnosis for men is around 68, about five years later than for women. By the time a man goes to the doctor about a lump, it has often been there for months.

Men with BRCA mutations have a much higher risk. A man with a BRCA2 mutation has up to a 1 in 10 chance of breast cancer in his lifetime, plus higher rates of prostate cancer and pancreatic cancer. That's why, when a family decides to test for BRCA, the boys have to get tested too. The mutation doesn't skip men.

If you are a guy reading this and you find something weird under your nipple, take it seriously. A lump behind a man's nipple is not "a weird lump" — it's a reason to see a doctor.

Myths vs. facts

When I started this project in grade 8, a lot of what I heard about breast cancer was wrong. Some of it was scary-wrong ("a lump always means cancer"); some was dangerous-wrong ("if no one in my family has had it, I don't need to worry"). Before we go any further, let's clear up the ones I hear most often.

Here are the myths one more time, in plain language, with the facts next to them:

- Myth: Only older women get breast cancer. Fact: Risk rises with age, but younger women can be diagnosed too. In The Bahamas, PAHO/WHO reported in 2026 that nearly half of diagnosed women are under 50.
- Myth: A lump always means cancer. Fact: Many lumps are benign, but a new or persistent lump should be evaluated — especially if it is clearly different from your normal.
- **Myth: Men can't get breast cancer.** Fact: They can. About 1 in 100 cases is in a man.
- **Myth: Wearing a bra or using deodorant causes cancer.** Fact: No study has ever shown this. Focus on real risks, not rumors.

- Myth: If no one in my family has had it, I am safe. Fact: Most breast cancers are not caused by an inherited high-risk mutation. Family history matters, but awareness and appropriate screening matter for everyone.
- Myth: Mammograms cause cancer. Fact: Mammography uses a low dose of radiation. For people in recommended screening groups, the proven benefit of detecting cancer earlier outweighs the small radiation risk.
- **Myth: Cancer is contagious.** Fact: You cannot catch cancer from hugging, kissing, or sharing food. You cannot give it to someone by sitting next to them in class.

Why early matters (already)

If you remember just one thing from this chapter, remember this: a cancer cell that is still inside the duct where it started is a very different problem from a cancer cell that has already traveled to the bone. The earlier we find it, the better the fight goes. That is the whole reason this book exists.

Chapter Two.

Types of Breast Cancer

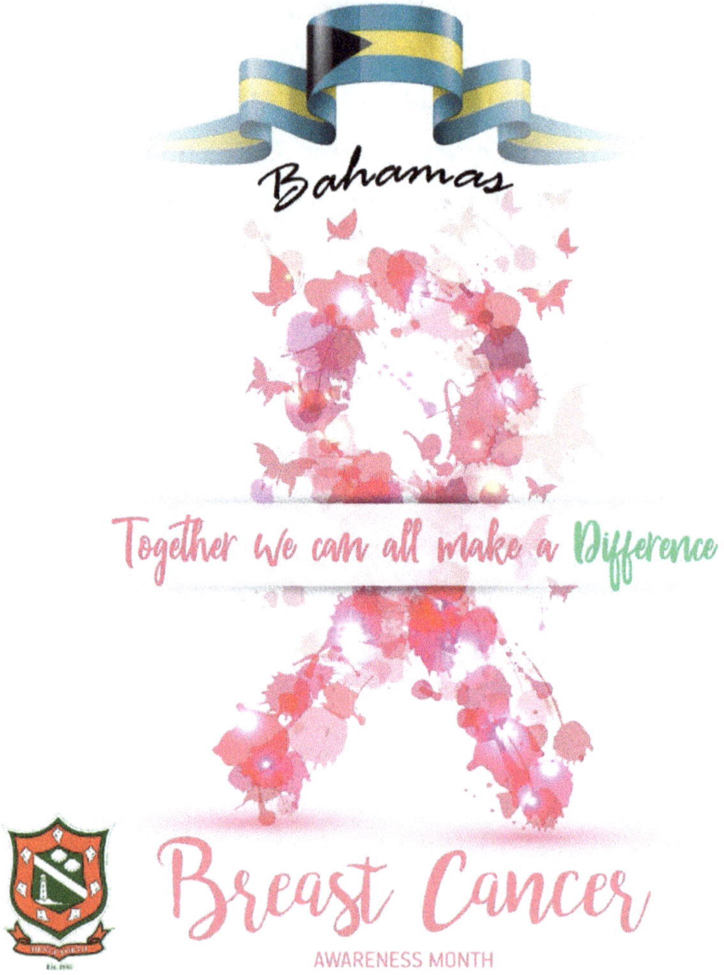

When I first started researching, I thought "breast cancer" was just one thing. It is not. It is actually a whole family of cancers that all start in the breast but behave differently, look different under a microscope, and need different treatments. Knowing the type is a huge part of figuring out the plan.

CUPCAKE CHECK — CHAPTER 2

Breast cancer is a family of diseases, not one disease.
Invasive vs. non-invasive matters.
ER, PR, HER2, grade, and other features help shape treatment.

Doctors group breast cancers a few different ways: by where the cancer started (ducts or lobules), by how much it has spread (non-invasive vs. invasive), by how the cells look under a microscope (the type), and by what molecules are on the cell's surface (the receptors). Each of those answers is a piece of the puzzle. Together, they tell the team what weapons will work.

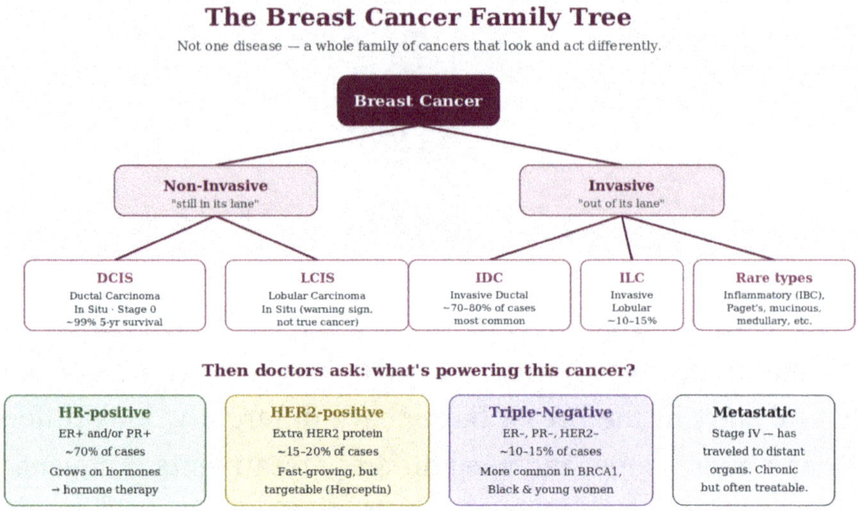

Figure 2.1 — The breast cancer family tree. All of these start in the breast but behave differently.

Let's go through the main ones.

Non-invasive: still in its lane

Non-invasive breast cancer means the cancer cells are there, but they haven't broken out of where they started. They are still inside the duct or the lobule. This is usually the earliest and most treatable form.

Ductal Carcinoma In Situ (DCIS) is the most common non-invasive type. "In situ" literally means "in place." The cancer cells are sitting inside a milk duct and have not punched through the duct wall. On its own, DCIS doesn't spread. But if it is left alone, some DCIS can become invasive over time, which is why doctors still treat it. About 1 in 5 new breast cancer diagnoses in the U.S. is DCIS — and nearly all of them are caught by mammograms, because you usually can't feel DCIS.

Lobular Carcinoma In Situ (LCIS) is less of a "cancer" and more of a warning sign. It means there are weird cells inside a lobule. LCIS usually doesn't turn into cancer itself, but having it raises the lifetime risk of getting breast cancer in the future — in either breast, not just the one where the LCIS was found. Women with LCIS are usually watched very closely, and sometimes take a hormone-blocking pill to lower the risk.

Invasive: out of its lane

Invasive means the cancer has broken out of the duct or the lobule and into the surrounding breast tissue. From there, it has the chance to reach lymph nodes and blood vessels.

Invasive Ductal Carcinoma (IDC) is by far the most common type of breast cancer — about 70 to 80 percent of all cases. It starts in a duct and then pushes out. Most lumps people feel during a self-exam turn out to be IDC when they are cancer.

Invasive Lobular Carcinoma (ILC) makes up about 10 to 15 percent of cases. It starts in a lobule. ILC is trickier because it tends to grow as a web of cells instead of one solid lump, which means it can be harder to feel and harder to see on a mammogram. Some women with ILC notice a thickening or "heaviness" on one side rather than a clear lump. That's a good reason to go by shape and feel overall — not just by whether you find a ball of tissue.

Rare types you should still know

Inflammatory Breast Cancer (IBC) is uncommon but serious. It may not form a lump. Instead, the breast can become red, warm, swollen, heavy, or dimpled like orange peel because cancer cells block lymph vessels in the skin. These changes can resemble infection. A rapidly changing red or swollen breast deserves prompt medical evaluation, especially if symptoms are not improving as expected with treatment for infection.

Paget's Disease of the Breast affects the skin of the nipple. It looks like a scaly, itchy rash, almost like eczema, on or around the nipple. It is usually a sign that there is a cancer inside the breast behind it. If a nipple rash doesn't heal with regular creams, get it checked.

Mucinous (colloid) carcinoma and medullary carcinoma are two rare subtypes of IDC that tend to be slower-growing and have better outcomes. Not every rare type is worse news.

Phyllodes tumors are rare growths that start in the connective tissue of the breast, not in the ducts. Most are benign, but some are malignant. They grow quickly, so any lump that changes size fast deserves a look.

Triple-Negative Breast Cancer (TNBC) is not about where the cancer started — it is about what the cells are missing. We will meet the three things they are "negative" for in the next section. TNBC is more common in younger women, in Black women, and in women with BRCA1 mutations. It tends to grow fast and is harder to treat because a lot of common drugs don't work on it. The good news: in the past few years, immunotherapy and newer chemo combinations have changed the outlook for TNBC patients in a real way.

HER2-positive cancers grow fast because the cells make too much of a protein called HER2 that tells them to divide. The good news: today, we have incredible drugs (like trastuzumab, brand name Herceptin, and newer ones like pertuzumab and trastuzumab deruxtecan) that lock onto HER2 and stop the cells. A diagnosis that was terrifying 30 years ago is much more treatable now because of these targeted therapies.

The three receptors doctors test for

When a cancer is diagnosed, doctors send a piece of it to a lab and ask three questions. The answers decide the whole treatment plan.

- **Is it ER-positive?** (ER = estrogen receptor) — estrogen is fueling the cancer.
- **Is it PR-positive?** (PR = progesterone receptor) — progesterone is fueling it.
- **Is it HER2-positive?** there's too much of the HER2 growth protein on the cells.

If the cancer is ER- or PR-positive, doctors can use hormone-blocking pills (like tamoxifen, or aromatase inhibitors like letrozole) to starve it. If it is HER2-positive, they can use targeted drugs. If it is triple-negative (all three are "no"), hormone and HER2 drugs won't help, and doctors rely more on chemotherapy and newer immunotherapy drugs like pembrolizumab.

It is the same cancer, but the type matters. A lot.

Grading: how "angry" do the cells look?

In addition to staging (how far the cancer has spread — see Chapter 3), every cancer gets a grade. A pathologist looks at the cells under a microscope and scores how normal or abnormal they look. Grade 1 cells look almost normal and tend to grow slowly. Grade 3 cells look wild and tend to grow quickly. Grade 2 is in between. Grade is useful because two cancers of the same stage can behave very differently depending on their grade.

The Ki-67 number

You may also see a number called Ki-67 on a pathology report. Ki-67 measures how many cells are actively dividing. A low Ki-67 (for example, 5%) means the cancer is sleepy; a high one (30% or more) means it's busy. Doctors use this to help decide how aggressive the treatment should be.

Talk to the pathology report

If someone you love is diagnosed, the pathology report can feel like a foreign language. Ask the doctor to walk through each part: the type (IDC/ILC/other), the grade (1–3), the receptor status (ER, PR, HER2), and the Ki-67 number. Those five pieces tell you the personality of the cancer.

Chapter Three.

Stages & Warning Signs

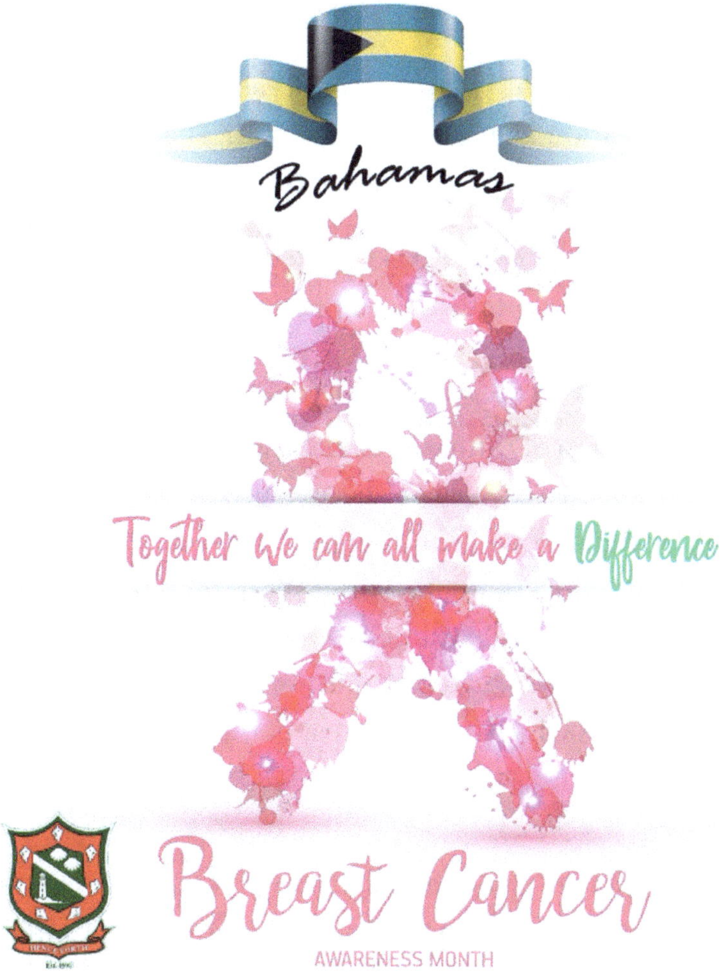

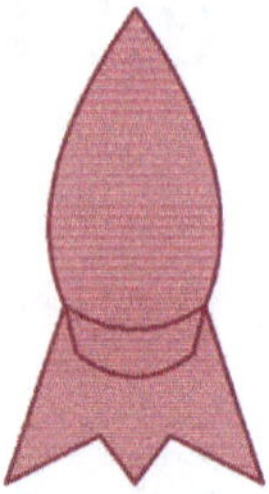

After doctors figure out what type of breast cancer someone has, the next big question is: how far has it gone? That's called staging, and it's basically the way we measure how serious a cancer is.

CUPCAKE CHECK — CHAPTER 3

Stage describes how far cancer has spread; modern staging also uses tumor biology.
A symptom is not a diagnosis — but persistent changes need evaluation.
Survival statistics describe groups, not an individual future.

The original version of this book asked, "Can Stage 1 breast cancer kill you?" I want to answer that honestly: yes, in rare cases, any cancer can be dangerous — but Stage 1 breast cancer is one of the most survivable cancers we know of. About 99 out of 100 women diagnosed at Stage 1 will still be alive five years later. That is an incredible number. The catch is that we have to actually catch it at Stage 1, which is what the whole rest of this book is really about.

The TNM system

Doctors stage cancer using three letters: T, N, and M. This system was developed by the American Joint Committee on Cancer, and it is used around the world so that a stage in Nassau means the same thing as a stage in New York.

- **T (Tumor)** — how big the main tumor is. T1 is 2 cm or less. T2 is 2–5 cm. T3 is over 5 cm. T4 is any size that has grown into the chest wall or the skin.
- **N (Nodes)** — whether the cancer has reached the lymph nodes, and how many. N0 means no nodes are involved. N1–N3 describes how many and how far.
- **M (Metastasis)** — whether it has traveled to far parts of the body like the bones, lungs, or liver. M0 is no spread. M1 is spread.

T and N get numbers (T1, T2, T3, T4), and M is either M0 (no spread) or M1 (spread). Doctors put those three letters together and use a chart to land on an overall stage from 0 to IV (4).

In 2018, the staging system got smarter. Now, in addition to T, N, and M, doctors also factor in the grade of the tumor and the receptor status. This is called the "prognostic stage group." A small ER-positive, low-grade tumor is a much gentler disease than a small triple-negative, high-grade tumor — and modern staging reflects that.

The stages, in plain English

Stage 0 usually refers to ductal carcinoma in situ (DCIS): abnormal cells are contained inside a milk duct and have not invaded surrounding breast tissue. DCIS is not included in the SEER localized invasive-cancer survival statistic.

Stage I generally describes a relatively small invasive cancer with little or no lymph-node involvement. The exact stage now also depends on tumor biology, grade, and receptor status.

Stage II usually means the cancer is larger and/or has reached a limited number of nearby lymph nodes, but has not spread to distant organs.

Stage III is locally advanced breast cancer. It can involve multiple nearby lymph nodes, the chest wall, or the skin, but there is no distant metastasis.

Stage IV means the breast cancer has spread to distant parts of the body, such as bone, liver, lung, or brain. It is called metastatic breast cancer. It is generally not considered curable, but it is treatable, and many people live meaningful lives for years with modern therapy.

SURVIVAL STATISTICS — USE THE RIGHT MAP

The American Cancer Society reports SEER survival by how far invasive cancer has spread, not by AJCC Stage I–IV. For women diagnosed in 2015–2021:

Localized: >99% 5-year relative survival
Regional: 87%
Distant: 32%
All SEER stages combined: 92%

A note on "5-year survival"

You will see "5-year relative survival" everywhere in cancer statistics. It compares people with a cancer diagnosis to similar people in the general population. It does not predict what will happen to one person, and it does not mean anyone "expires" at five years. Treatment keeps improving, and factors such as age, tumor biology, response to treatment, access to care, and overall health all matter.

Warning signs — know what to look for

Most of the time, the person who first notices breast cancer is not a doctor. It is the woman herself, her partner, or a family member. That is why knowing the warning signs matters.

The most common sign is a new lump. Cancer lumps usually feel hard, uneven, and don't hurt to touch. But some cancers don't make a lump at all.

Other warning signs include:

- Skin dimpling that looks like the peel of an orange
- A nipple that suddenly pulls inward (inverted) when it didn't before
- Fluid coming from the nipple that is not breast milk — especially if it has blood in it
- Redness, rash, warmth, or flaky skin on the breast or nipple that won't heal
- Swelling where part of the breast looks bigger or a different shape
- A lump in the armpit (remember: breast tissue reaches into the underarm)
- Pain in one spot that won't go away
- Thickening or hardening in one area, even without a clear lump (this can be a sign of lobular cancer)
- An area that just "doesn't feel right" — trust that instinct

One symptom on its own usually doesn't mean cancer. Lumps especially are almost always something less scary (like a cyst or a normal change during a period). But any change that sticks around for more than a couple of weeks is a reason to see a doctor. Not someday. Soon.

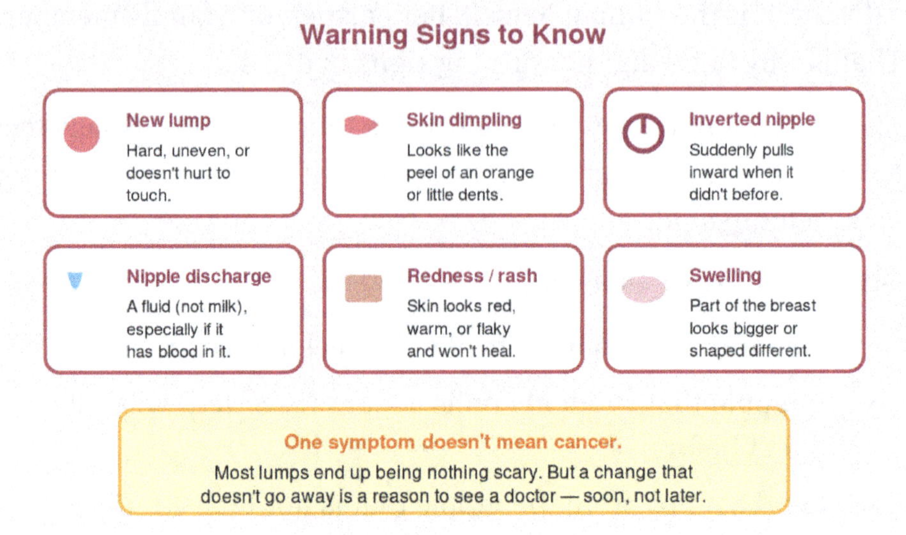

Figure 3.3 — Common warning signs. One symptom doesn't mean cancer — but changes that last are worth a visit.

When to call the doctor — a flowchart

If you're not sure whether something you notice is worth a call, this flowchart can help. It isn't a replacement for a doctor's advice — it's a simple "how urgent?" guide.

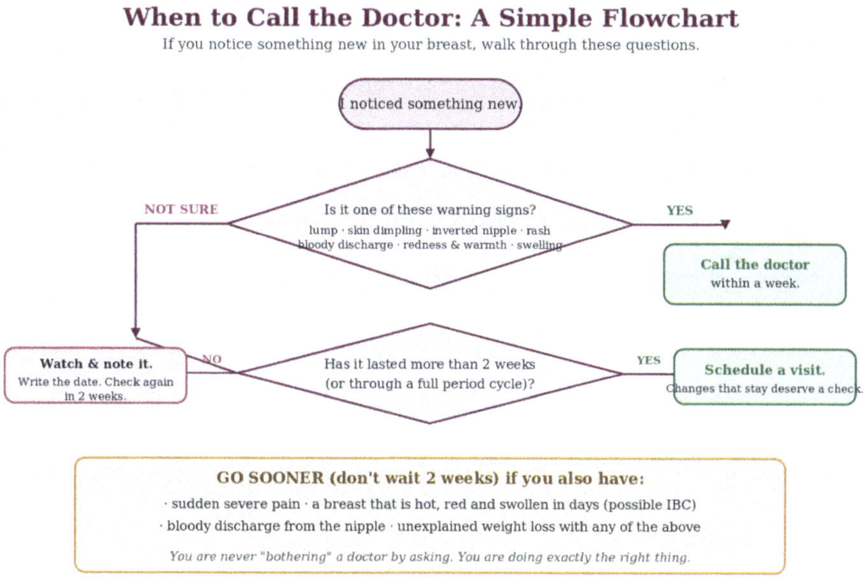

Figure 3.4 — A simple flowchart for deciding when to book an appointment.

What happens at the appointment

If you go to a doctor with a breast concern, here's what usually happens. First, the doctor will ask questions — how long has it been there, has it changed, any family history. Then they'll do a clinical breast exam, feeling both breasts and the lymph nodes under your arms and above your collarbone. They may order imaging — a mammogram if you're over 40, or an ultrasound if you're younger because young breast tissue is dense and ultrasounds see through it better. If anything looks suspicious, the next step is a biopsy, where a small sample of the tissue is taken with a needle. The biopsy is the only way to know for sure whether something is cancer. It usually takes a few days to a week to get results — the hardest waiting room of your life. Most biopsies come back normal.

The rule my mom taught me

"If something is there, and it wasn't there last month, and it still hasn't gone away this month — get it checked." That's it. That's the rule. You don't need to diagnose it yourself. You just need to show up.

Chapter Four.

Genes, Risks & BRCA

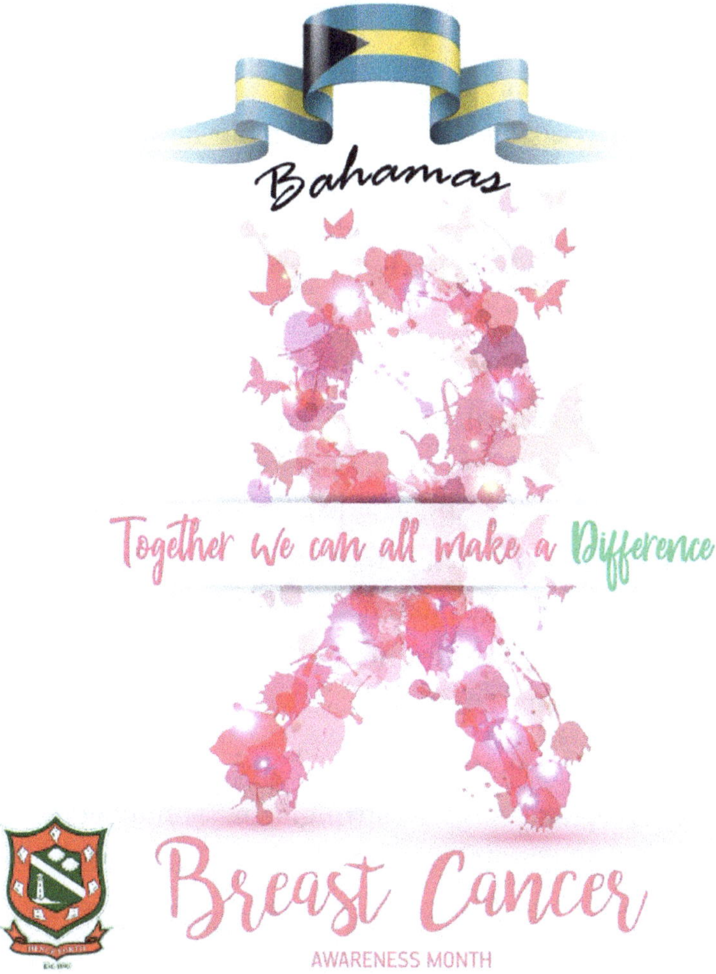

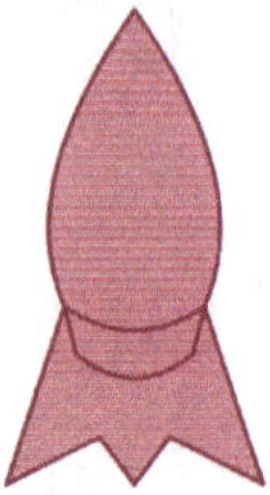

When people hear that a woman has breast cancer, the first question they often ask is, "Does it run in her family?" The answer is sometimes yes, and it is a bigger deal than people think.

> **CUPCAKE CHECK – CHAPTER 4**
>
> Most breast cancers are not explained by inherited high-risk mutations.
> BRCA1/BRCA2 are especially important in Bahamian breast-cancer research.
> Genetic testing is most useful when paired with counseling and a plan.

About 5 to 10 percent of all breast cancers are hereditary — which means they come from a gene the person was born with, passed down from a parent. The other 90 to 95 percent are what doctors call sporadic, which basically means "it just happened." Both kinds are real. Both can be beaten. But the hereditary ones are the ones you can actually plan around, because you can find out about them before they cause trouble.

That 5–10% number is an average — and averages lie in places where breast cancer runs strong. In some communities (including ours, in The Bahamas), the real fraction is closer to 1 in 4 patients. We'll meet that number again in Chapter 6.

Meet BRCA1 and BRCA2

Inside every one of your cells, you have two genes with really important jobs: BRCA1 and BRCA2. Their names stand for "BReast CAncer gene 1" and "BReast CAncer gene 2," but that's a little misleading. These genes don't cause breast cancer. They actually prevent it.

BRCA1 and BRCA2 are what scientists call tumor suppressor genes. Their job is to find DNA damage in a cell and fix it before the cell can turn into cancer. They are the spell-checkers of the cell.

But sometimes, a person is born with a mutation — a tiny typo — in one of those genes. The spell-checker stops working. Over a lifetime, tiny DNA mistakes build up in breast and ovary cells because nobody is catching them. That's why women with a BRCA mutation have a much higher risk of breast and ovarian cancer.

BRCA mutations are inherited. If your mom has one, you have a 50% chance of having it too. So do your siblings, your aunts, and your cousins. That's why BRCA testing is considered a family project, not an individual one. One person's result tells a whole extended family something important about themselves.

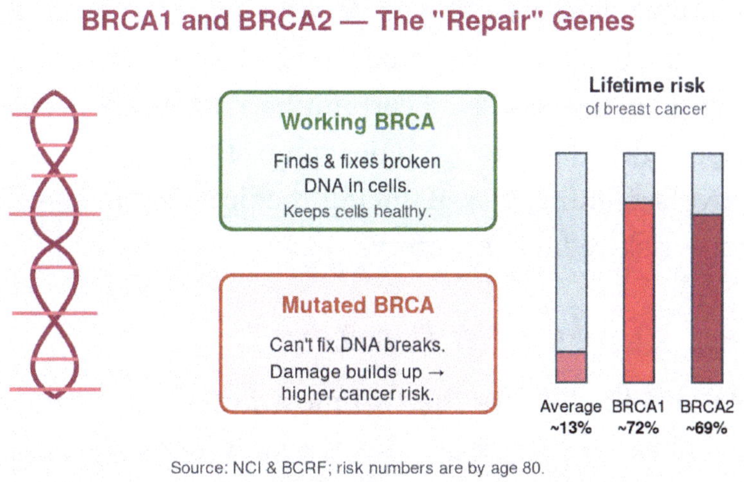

Figure 4.1 — BRCA1 & BRCA2 normally repair DNA damage; a mutation can dramatically raise cancer risk.

How much higher is the risk?

The numbers are sobering:

- **An average woman has about a 13 percent lifetime risk of breast cancer.**
- **A woman with a BRCA1 mutation has about a 55–72 percent lifetime risk.**
- **A woman with a BRCA2 mutation has about a 45–69 percent lifetime risk.**
- **BRCA mutations also raise the risk of ovarian cancer (up to about 44% for BRCA1 and 17% for BRCA2).**

And BRCA isn't only a "female gene." Men with BRCA mutations have higher rates of breast cancer (yes, really), prostate cancer, and pancreatic cancer. So when a family is checking for BRCA, the boys need to get tested too.

A BRCA mutation is not a diagnosis of cancer. It is a high-risk signal. More than 60% of women who inherit a harmful BRCA1 or BRCA2 change are expected to develop breast cancer during their lifetime, but risk is not certainty. Knowing about a mutation can open the door to genetic counseling, earlier and more intensive screening, risk-reducing medication, and — for some people — risk-reducing surgery.

Other genes that matter

BRCA1 and BRCA2 are the two most famous hereditary breast cancer genes, but they are not the only ones. Genetic testing panels today check for many others, including:

- **PALB2** — a gene that partners with BRCA2. A mutation in PALB2 raises breast cancer risk to roughly 35–50%. Found in Trinidad & Tobago in notable numbers.
- **CHEK2** — a gene that slows cells down when DNA is damaged. Mutations raise risk by roughly 2× the general population.
- **ATM** — another DNA repair gene; mutations raise risk by roughly 2–3×.
- **TP53** — mutations cause Li-Fraumeni syndrome, a rare condition that raises risk for many cancers, often at young ages.
- **PTEN** — mutations cause Cowden syndrome, which raises risk for breast, thyroid, and uterine cancers.
- **CDH1** — raises risk for invasive lobular cancer and gastric cancer.

None of these numbers is a sentence. They are information that lets families plan. And the list keeps growing — gene testing labs now look at 30 or more genes at once, instead of just two.

Reading a family pedigree

Genetic counselors build a picture of a family using a diagram called a pedigree. Squares are boys and men; circles are girls and women. Filled-in shapes are people who have had cancer. Once you draw it out, patterns jump off the page.

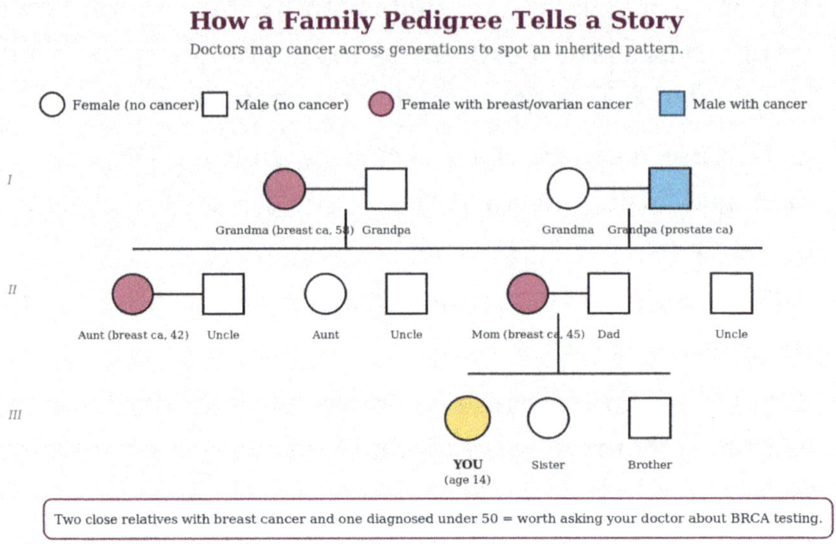

Figure 4.2 — A sample family pedigree. Two close relatives with breast cancer, one diagnosed before 50 = worth asking about BRCA testing.

When a genetic counselor looks at a pedigree, here are the red flags that suggest an inherited mutation:

- Breast cancer in two or more close relatives on the same side of the family
- Any relative diagnosed before age 50
- Ovarian cancer in any close relative, at any age
- A male relative with breast cancer
- A relative with both breast and ovarian cancer
- Bilateral (both breasts) breast cancer in one person
- Triple-negative breast cancer before age 60
- Pancreatic or aggressive prostate cancer in multiple relatives
- Ashkenazi Jewish, Bahamian, or certain other founder-mutation ancestry

If a family has any of these patterns, it's worth asking a doctor or genetic counselor about testing.

Who should think about getting tested?

You don't need a genetic test just because you watched a movie about breast cancer. But if any of these apply, a doctor might recommend one:

- **A mother, sister, or daughter who had breast cancer, especially before age 50**
- **Two or more close relatives with breast or ovarian cancer**
- **A male relative with breast cancer**
- **Being of Ashkenazi Jewish descent, or (as we'll see in Chapter 6) Bahamian descent**
- **A relative who has already tested positive for a BRCA mutation**

Testing is usually a simple blood test or cheek swab. And knowing you have a BRCA mutation doesn't mean you will get cancer. It means you can be watched closely, screened earlier, and, if you want, take steps to lower the risk — including preventive medications and, in some cases, preventive surgery.

What happens if a test is positive?

If someone tests positive for BRCA1 or BRCA2, a genetic counselor will help them make a plan. Options usually include:

- Starting breast MRI and mammograms at age 25–30, every year
- Consider risk-reducing medications like tamoxifen or raloxifene

- Consider risk-reducing mastectomy (preventive breast removal) — a personal decision
- Risk-reducing removal of the ovaries and fallopian tubes, usually between ages 35–45 after childbearing
- Sharing the result with close relatives so they can be tested too

No one option is right for everyone. Some women choose intensive screening; others choose preventive surgery. Both are valid.

Other things that change the risk

Some risk factors we can't change: being a woman, getting older, having your period very early (before 12), hitting menopause very late (after 55), and dense breast tissue. Some risk factors we can change: drinking a lot of alcohol, not being physically active, being very overweight after menopause, smoking, and in some cases, long-term use of hormone replacement therapy.

Risk Factors You Can and Can't Change

Knowing the difference helps you focus your energy where it matters.

CAN'T CHANGE

- Being female (~99% of cases)
- Getting older (risk climbs with age)
- Genetics (BRCA1, BRCA2, PALB2...)
- Family history of breast cancer
- Starting periods early (before 12)
- Menopause late (after 55)
- Dense breast tissue
- Past chest radiation (e.g. for Hodgkin's lymphoma as a child)
- Ancestry (e.g. Bahamian, Ashkenazi)

CAN CHANGE

- Drinking alcohol → lower or avoid
- Smoking / vaping → quit
- Being inactive → aim for 150 min/wk
- Weight after menopause → keep stable, healthy range
- Long-term hormone replacement therapy → discuss risks with doctor
- Breastfeeding if possible → lowers risk slightly
- Skipping screenings → show up!
- Silence in the family → talk about who has had what, and when

Most women who get breast cancer don't have a clear risk factor — that's why awareness matters for everyone.

Figure 4.3 — Breast cancer risk factors divided into "can change" and "can't change." Focus your energy where it counts.

How much does each thing matter?

Not all risk factors are equal. Here's a rough sense, based on major studies:

- Being female: ~100× the risk of being male
- Being older: risk doubles roughly every 10 years from age 30 to 80
- BRCA1 mutation: 5–6× the average lifetime risk
- First-degree relative with breast cancer: ~2× the risk
- Dense breast tissue: ~1.2–2× the risk
- Alcohol (3+ drinks per day): ~1.5× the risk
- Being overweight after menopause: ~1.3× the risk
- Physical inactivity: ~1.2× the risk
- Long-term hormone replacement therapy: ~1.2–1.3× the risk

The biggest thing you can control at any age is your health habits. Regular exercise, eating a lot of vegetables, not smoking, and keeping alcohol low don't make you bulletproof, but they do lower the odds. And they help with every other part of your health too.

If you're a teen reading this

You don't need to be worrying about mammograms yet. But two things you can do right now that matter for life: (1) talk to an older family member this week and ask, "Has anyone in our family had breast, ovarian, prostate, or pancreatic cancer? At what age?" Write it down. (2) Build health habits you actually enjoy — not to be "healthy" but to be strong. Exercise, sleep, cooking real food, skipping alcohol. These stack for decades.

Chapter Five.

Breast Awareness & Early Detection

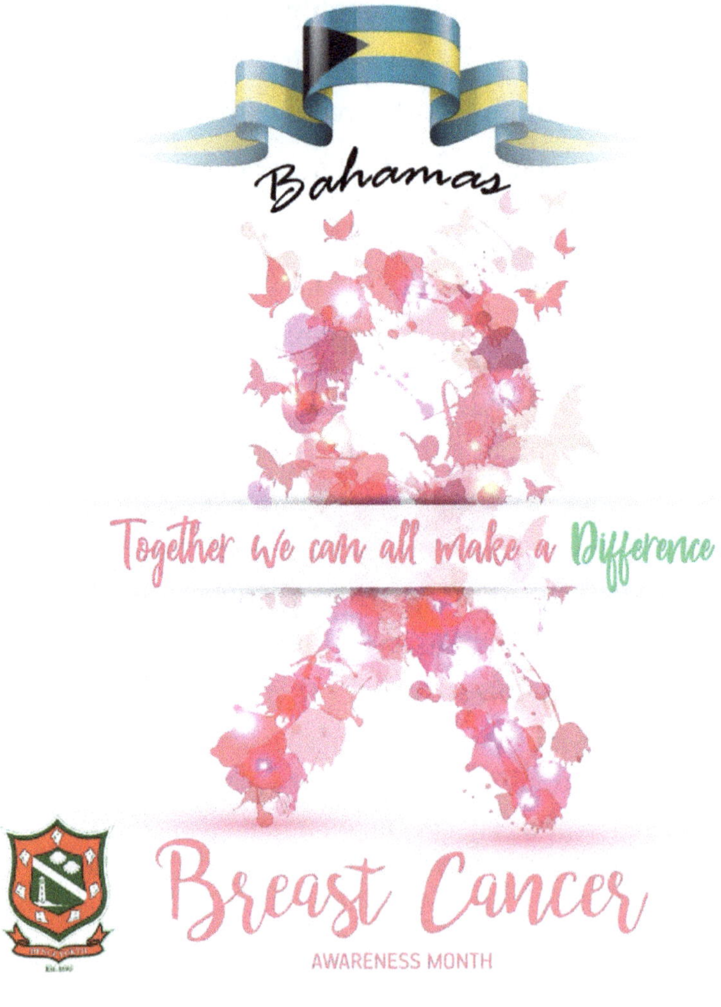

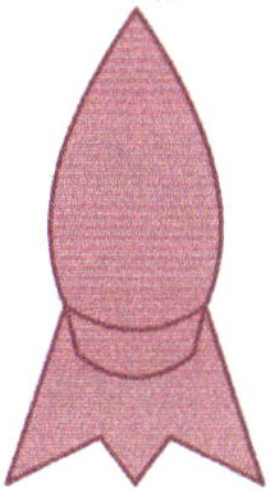

This might be the most useful chapter in the whole book. Early evaluation and recommended screening can find some cancers before they spread. In current U.S. SEER data, 5-year relative survival is greater than 99% for localized invasive breast cancer and about 32% for distant disease.

CUPCAKE CHECK – CHAPTER 5

Know what is normal for your body.
Report a new or persistent change promptly.
Follow a screening plan based on age, risk, and current guidance.

There are three practical pieces to early detection: know what is normal for your body, report new or persistent changes promptly, and follow a screening plan that fits your age and risk. Mammography is the main screening test for people at average risk.

Know your normal (breast awareness)

Something changed since the first version of this book. For a long time, doctors taught a strict monthly "breast self-exam" – the same moves, every month, same day of your cycle. Recent research (from the American Cancer Society and others) found that a strict monthly routine didn't actually save more lives.

So the advice shifted to something called breast awareness. It means: know what your breasts normally look and feel like, so you will notice if something changes. That's it.

Getting to know your normal is still done the same way as a self-exam — by looking and feeling. The difference is that you don't have to be perfect about the schedule. You just have to pay attention.

You do not need a rigid monthly self-exam schedule. Some people find an occasional look-and-feel check useful simply because it helps them notice what is normal. The goal is awareness, not perfect technique or a calendar ritual.

Here is a version of the five-step check you can use anytime:

- **Step 1:** Stand in front of a mirror with your shoulders straight and your hands on your hips. Look. Are your breasts their usual size, shape, and color? Any swelling, dimpling, redness, or rash?
- **Step 2:** Raise your arms above your head. Look for the same changes. Raised arms pull the breast tissue tighter against the chest and make changes easier to spot.
- Step 3: Notice the nipples. A new inversion, skin change, or spontaneous discharge — especially clear or bloody discharge from one side — is worth telling a healthcare professional about. Discharge can have many benign causes, so this is a reason to check, not a reason to panic.
- **Step 4:** Lie down. Use the pads of your three middle fingers to feel each breast. Use small, overlapping circles and cover the whole area — from your collarbone to the top of your belly, and from the middle of your chest into your armpit. Use light, medium, and firm pressure in each spot.

- **Step 5:** Repeat Step 4 in the shower, while your skin is wet and soapy. A lot of women find it easier to notice changes this way.

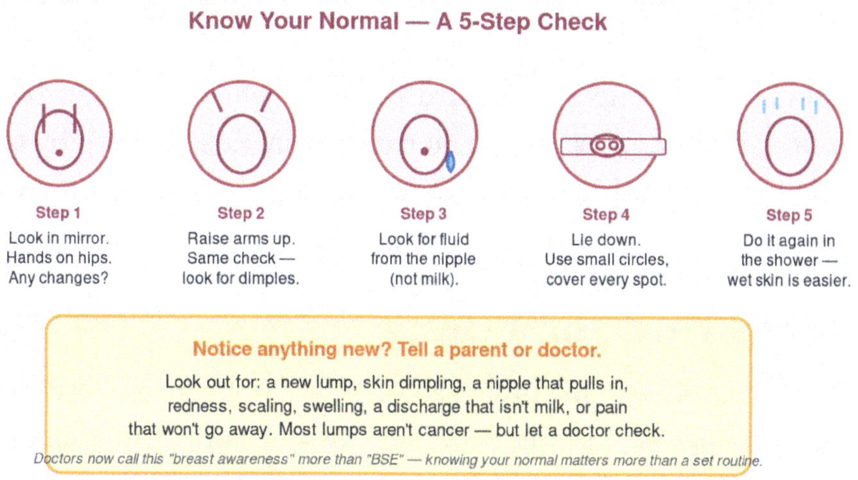

Figure 5.1 — A 5-step breast awareness check you can do anytime.

Common things you might feel — and what they usually mean

When you do a self-check, you will feel things. Breasts are not smooth organs. They have natural ridges, lumps, and soft spots. Here are the most common non-cancer things:

- **Fibrocystic changes** — lumpy, rope-like texture, sometimes tender, usually worse before a period. Very common, not cancer.
- **Cysts** — fluid-filled round bumps, often tender, that can change with your cycle. Sometimes doctors drain them with a needle.

- **Fibroadenomas** — solid, smooth, rubbery lumps that move easily under the skin. Most common in women under 30. Almost always benign.
- **Lipomas** — soft fat lumps that feel squishy. Almost never cancer.

Some breast cancers are hard or fixed, but others can be soft, round, tender, or painful. You cannot diagnose a lump by touch. The important thing is whether it is new or different for you — that is when a clinician and imaging can help.

If you find something

Do not panic — many breast changes are not cancer — but do not use a two-week waiting rule for a new or concerning change. A new lump, persistent thickening, skin or nipple change, or unusual discharge deserves medical advice promptly, especially if it is worsening or clearly different from your normal.

When you do call the doctor, here are the things worth saying: how big it feels, where it is, whether it moves when you push it, whether it hurts, and how long it has been there. Write the date on a calendar. That date is more useful than any description.

Clinical exams

A clinical breast exam is when a doctor or nurse does a breast check during a regular physical. They are trained to feel for subtle things you might miss. If your pediatrician or family doctor doesn't do one, it is okay to ask.

A clinical breast exam can be useful when someone has a symptom, a new change, or higher-than-average risk. The American Cancer Society does not recommend routine clinical breast exams as a stand-alone screening test for average-risk women. If something feels different, a clinician can examine it and decide whether imaging is needed.

Mammograms — the gold standard

A mammogram is a special X-ray of the breast. It can find lumps up to two years before you could feel them yourself. That is a huge head start.

A mammogram works by squishing the breast between two plates so the X-ray can see through the tissue. The squish takes a few seconds per view. It is uncomfortable, yes. But it is very safe, and the radiation dose is tiny — less than a round-trip flight from Nassau to New York.

For average-risk women, two widely used U.S. guidance sets are:

- American Cancer Society: ages 40–44 may choose yearly mammography.
- American Cancer Society: ages 45–54 should have yearly mammography.
- American Cancer Society: age 55 and older may switch to every 2 years or continue yearly screening while in good health.
- USPSTF: biennial mammography from ages 40–74 for average-risk women. People with BRCA-related risk, prior chest radiation, previous breast cancer, or other high-risk features need an individualized plan that can start earlier and may include MRI.

Mammograms are not perfect. They can lead to callbacks, extra imaging, false positives, and sometimes overdiagnosis, but screening mammography lowers breast-cancer mortality. The balance of benefits and harms depends on age and risk, which is why screening schedules differ slightly between major organizations.

3D mammograms and other new imaging

Most centers now use digital mammograms, which store the images on a computer. Some also offer 3D mammograms (also called tomosynthesis), where the X-ray takes pictures from multiple angles and builds a layered image. 3D mammograms are especially helpful for women with dense breast tissue — they find more cancers and give fewer false alarms.

If you have dense breast tissue, your doctor may also recommend supplemental screening — a whole-breast ultrasound, or a breast MRI. Dense tissue is the radiologist's version of snow on the windshield: it hides things. Extra tools help see through it.

What to expect at a mammogram

If you've never had one, here's what happens. You go to the imaging center, change into a gown from the waist up, and a technologist (almost always a woman) brings you into a room with a tall machine. She helps you position one breast on a flat plate; another plate comes down from above and compresses it for a few seconds while the X-ray is taken. Two views per breast is standard — one top-to-bottom, one side angle. The whole visit takes about 20 minutes. You can go back to work after.

Most results are normal. If the radiologist wants a closer look at something, they call you back for extra images or an ultrasound. About 10% of women get called back for a second look, and of those, most are still normal. A callback is not a diagnosis.

MRI, ultrasound, and other screening tools

Breast MRI uses magnets and radio waves (no ionizing radiation) to make detailed images. It is more sensitive than mammography, but it can also create more false alarms. MRI is commonly added for people at very high risk, such as many BRCA carriers. Dense breasts alone do not automatically mean MRI or ultrasound is required; the decision should consider overall risk and local guidance.

Ultrasound uses sound waves to see through tissue. It's especially useful for young women with dense breasts, for distinguishing solid lumps from fluid-filled cysts, and for guiding a biopsy needle.

Blood tests cannot yet reliably screen for early breast cancer in healthy people, but new "liquid biopsy" tests that look for tiny fragments of tumor DNA in the blood are in active research. That is an area to watch over the next five to ten years.

Screening timeline at a glance

Here is the short version of what screening should look like at each stage of life for most women:

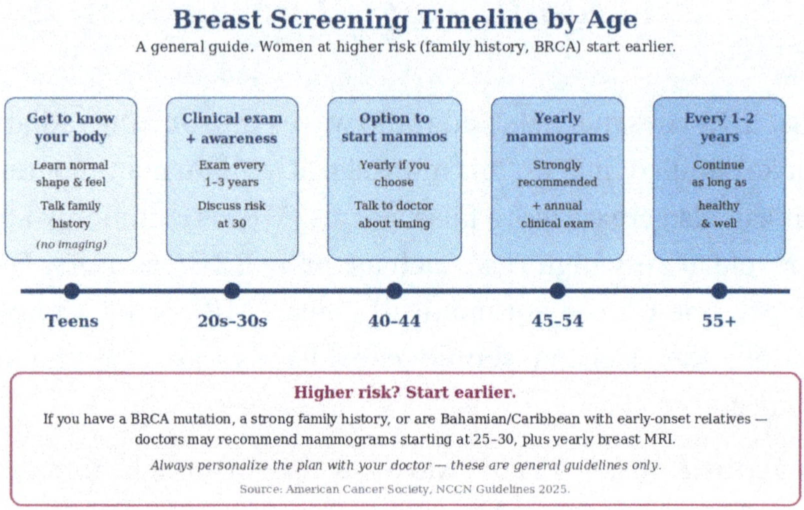

Figure 5.2 — General screening timeline by age. High-risk women start earlier and add MRI.

The 3 steps, for anyone in a rush

1. Know your normal. 2. See a doctor if something changes. 3. Get screened on schedule. That's it. That's the whole game plan.

Chapter Six.

The Caribbean Breast Cancer Story: The Bahamas & Beyond

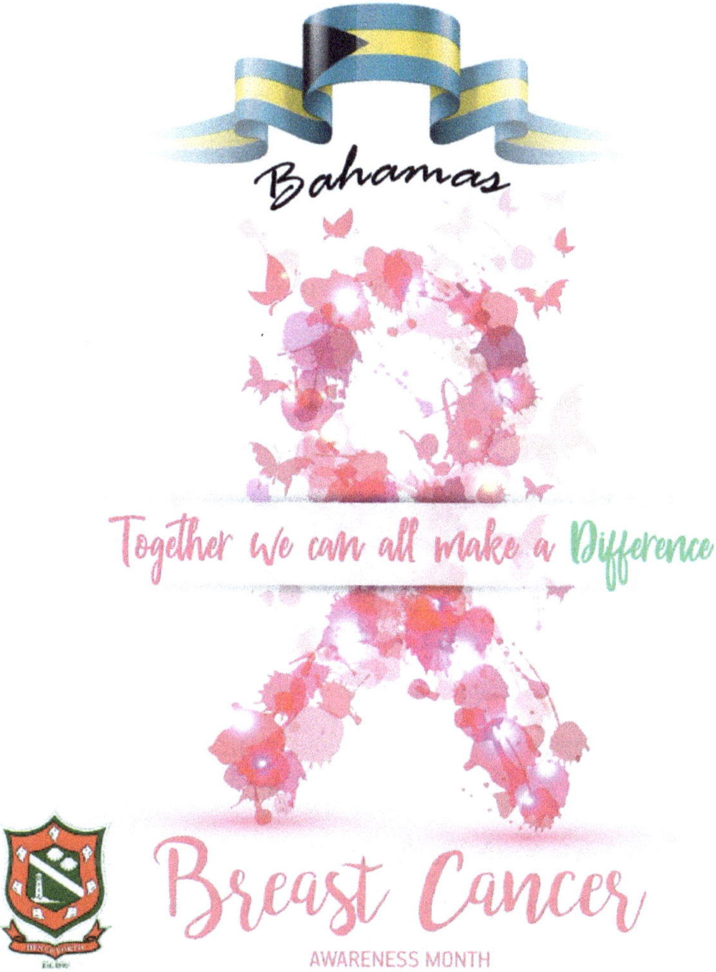

This is the chapter that made me want to turn this project into a real book — because the Bahamian story is not a footnote. It is one of the reasons this book needs to exist.

> **CUPCAKE CHECK — CHAPTER 6**
>
> The Bahamian breast-cancer story includes unusually important hereditary risk.
>
> Nearly half of diagnosed Bahamian women are under 50, according to PAHO/WHO in 2026.
>
> Access, timing, treatment, genetics, and geography all affect outcomes.

I live in The Bahamas. When I started researching breast cancer, I expected to find articles about America and Europe, because that's where most of the money and research is. I didn't expect to find my own country at the top of a list I didn't want us to be on.

A number I couldn't stop thinking about

Bahamian breast-cancer research found an unusually high prevalence of inherited BRCA1/BRCA2 mutations among women who had breast cancer.

The numbers come from landmark Bahamian studies. In a 2011 study of 214 unselected Bahamian women with invasive breast cancer, 23% carried one of six BRCA1 founder mutations. A 2014 expanded analysis of the same 214-patient series found BRCA1 or BRCA2 mutations in 58 women — 27% — and reported that 92% of mutation carriers had one of seven founder mutations. These were studies of women who already had breast cancer, not a statement that 27% of all Bahamian women carry BRCA mutations.

That remains an extraordinary finding. NCI estimates inherited BRCA1/BRCA2 changes occur in roughly 1 in 400 to 1 in 800 people in the general population outside groups with known founder mutations. The Bahamian research shows why genetic counseling and testing deserve special attention here — especially after a breast or ovarian cancer diagnosis or when there is a strong family history.

This is not a small piece of trivia. It is one of the most important pieces of breast-cancer information our families can know — but it has to be interpreted correctly and with genetic counseling.

BAHAMAS FOCUS — WHAT THE 2026 PAHO/WHO ASSESSMENT SAID

Cancer control in The Bahamas was under comprehensive review in 2026. PAHO/WHO highlighted three facts that belong in every national conversation:

Breast cancer is the leading cause of cancer-related death among women in The Bahamas.
Nearly half of women diagnosed are under age 50.
Almost half present at an advanced stage.

The hopeful side is that founder mutations are easier to target with focused testing. Research in unaffected Bahamian women has also shown that family history can help identify people who may benefit from genetic counseling and testing. The point is not to make everyone afraid; it is to make useful information easier to reach.

Why the whole Caribbean is at higher risk

The Bahamas is not alone. Across the Caribbean, breast-cancer outcomes are shaped by a mix of biology, screening access, diagnosis timing, treatment availability, health-system capacity, and social barriers. The pattern is not identical on every island, so I do not want to flatten the region into one statistic.

Three patterns make our region different:

- Younger diagnosis matters in our region. In The Bahamas, PAHO/WHO reported in 2026 that nearly half of women diagnosed with breast cancer are under 50.
- Late and advanced presentation remains a major challenge. The same 2026 PAHO/WHO assessment reported that almost half of Bahamian breast-cancer cases present at an advanced stage.
- Tumor biology also matters. Triple-negative breast cancer is more common in Black women, and hereditary mutations are an especially important part of the Bahamian story.

THE CARIBBEAN STORY AT A GLANCE

The region is diverse, but three recurring questions help organize the chapter:

Can people reach screening, imaging, pathology, and follow-up early enough?
Do patients have access to the treatments their tumor biology requires?
Are hereditary-cancer services available to families who may benefit from them?

A closer look by country

The Bahamas — historic research found BRCA1/BRCA2 mutations in 27% of a 214-patient breast-cancer series. In 2026,

PAHO/WHO also reported that nearly half of diagnosed women are under 50 and almost half present at an advanced stage.

Jamaica — breast cancer is a major women's health burden. Screening access and timely follow-up outside major urban centers remain important parts of the conversation.

Trinidad & Tobago — hereditary-cancer research has identified pathogenic variants across BRCA1, BRCA2, PALB2 and other genes, reinforcing the value of genetic services across the Caribbean.

Barbados — breast cancer remains a significant public-health challenge, with continued emphasis on earlier detection and access to oncology care.

Haiti — access to screening, pathology, treatment, and continuity of care is limited for many patients, making partnerships and health-system capacity especially important.

Dominican Republic, Cuba, and Puerto Rico — cancer systems and screening capacity differ substantially across these settings. The lesson is that "the Caribbean" is not one health system; every country needs data and solutions that fit its own population.

Why are the numbers worse here?

This part made me really sad when I first learned it, because most of the reasons are things we can change.

- Uneven screening access. Mammography, diagnostic imaging, pathology, and follow-up are not equally available across every island or community.

- Late diagnosis. Fear, cost, travel, limited capacity, and gaps in screening or follow-up can all contribute to cancers being found at a more advanced stage.
- Access to treatment. Modern targeted therapies, immunotherapies, radiation services, surgery, and supportive care may be harder to access or finance in smaller health systems.
- Genetic services. The Bahamas has a strong scientific case for wider access to genetic counseling and appropriate testing, but testing should be connected to counseling, surveillance, and care.
- **Stigma.** In some families, cancer still isn't talked about openly. That silence delays care.
- Workforce and geography. Small-island health systems must cover many communities across water, which can make specialist access, treatment schedules, and follow-up harder.
- Biology and inequity can overlap. Younger diagnosis, triple-negative disease, hereditary risk, late presentation, and access barriers can compound one another.

What we can actually do

This is what gives me hope: the research on Bahamian women's risk means we know what to look for. A targeted genetic testing program in The Bahamas could identify BRCA carriers before they ever get cancer, giving them screening, preventive options, and a real chance. Groups like the Sister Sister Breast Cancer Support Group, the Cancer Society of The Bahamas, and international partners are pushing hard for this.

If you are a Bahamian woman — or the daughter of one — these are worth doing:

- **Ask about your family history.** A mother, aunt, or grandmother who had breast or ovarian cancer (especially before age 50) is a big signal.
- **Ask a doctor** whether BRCA testing makes sense for your family.
- **Start breast awareness young.** In the Caribbean, this matters even more because of younger diagnosis ages.
- Ask for a risk-based screening plan. A strong family history or known pathogenic variant can change when screening starts and which tests are used; this should be decided with a qualified clinician or genetics team.
- **Support local breast cancer organizations.** Their work is literally saving Caribbean lives. Fundraisers, donations, and volunteer hours matter.
- **Talk about it.** If your auntie had breast cancer, let your cousins know. If your mom was diagnosed young, tell your daughters. Breaking silence in one family changes many lives.

Bahamian voices that are changing the story

The fight against breast cancer in The Bahamas isn't just doctors and researchers. It is survivors and advocates. It is the women of the Sister Sister Breast Cancer Support Group, founded by the late Mrs. Andrea Sweeting, who turned personal loss into a national support network. It is the Fox Foundation, which provides free breast exams during awareness month. It is the Cancer Society of The Bahamas, which fundraises for patients who could not otherwise afford treatment. It is the oncology nurses at the Princess Margaret Hospital, who sit with women through chemo that takes all day. And it is the teachers, church leaders, and student council members who pick up pink ribbons every October and refuse to let the conversation die when November comes.

There is a place for you in this, too.

Be the one who breaks the silence

At the next family gathering, you get one conversation. Ask who has had cancer — breast, ovarian, prostate, pancreatic, or colon — and at what age. Write it on your phone. That little list is the single most useful piece of medical information you will ever carry.

Chapter Seven.

Treatments & Integrative Care

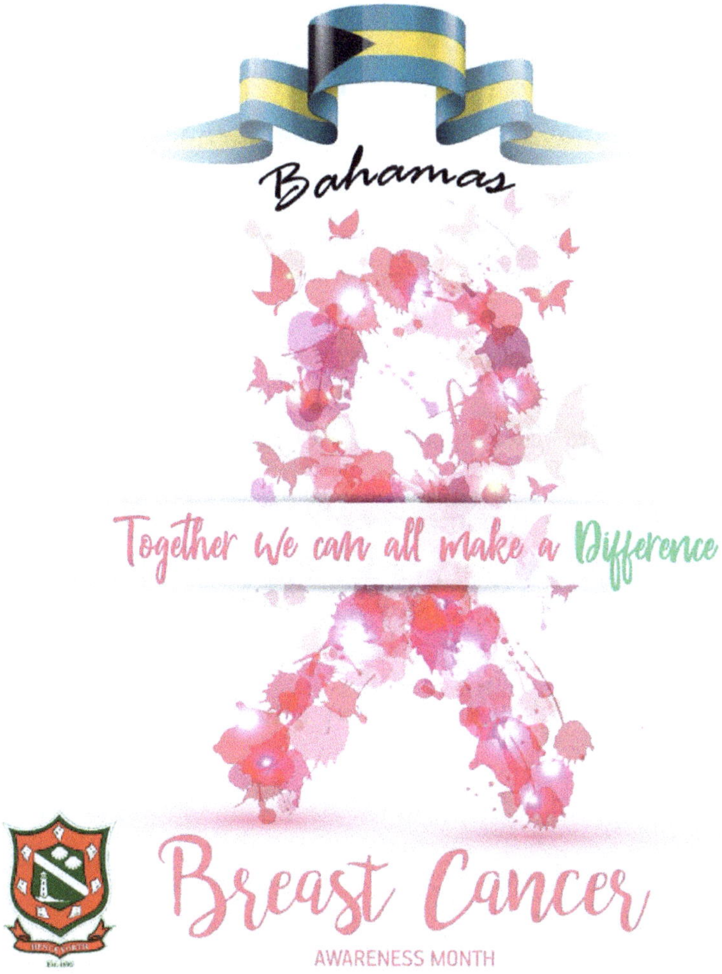

If someone is diagnosed with breast cancer, the treatment depends on so many things — the type of cancer, the stage, the receptors, age, general health, and sometimes what the patient wants. There is no one treatment. There is a plan.

> **CUPCAKE CHECK – CHAPTER 7**
>
> There is no single breast-cancer treatment plan.
> Surgery, radiation, and systemic therapies are combined according to tumor biology and stage.
> Complementary care should support – never replace – evidence-based cancer treatment.

In most cases, the plan combines two or more of the treatments in this chapter. A treatment plan is built by an "oncology team" — usually a medical oncologist (the chemo doctor), a surgical oncologist or breast surgeon, a radiation oncologist, and a pathologist. They look at every detail and design a course just for that patient.

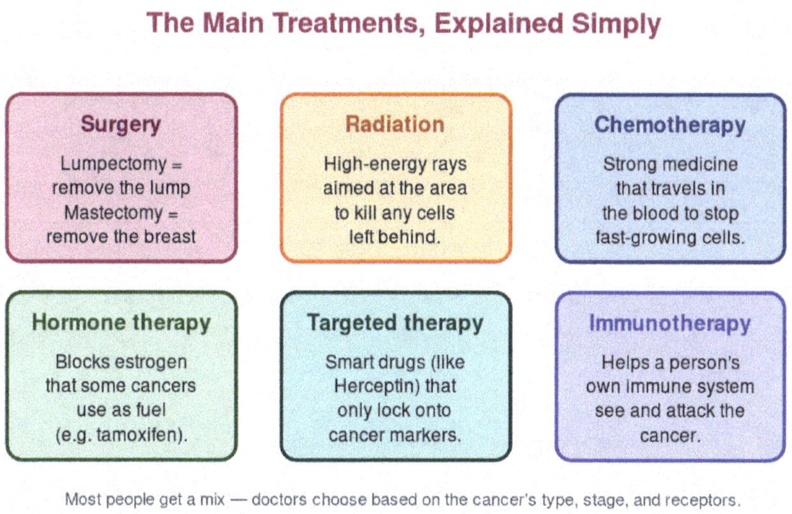

Figure 7.1 — The main treatments doctors use to fight breast cancer. Most plans combine several.

The treatment journey, step by step

A typical early-stage journey looks like the timeline below. It is a lot when you read it all at once, but in real life it unfolds over months. Each step has its own appointments, choices, and recovery time.

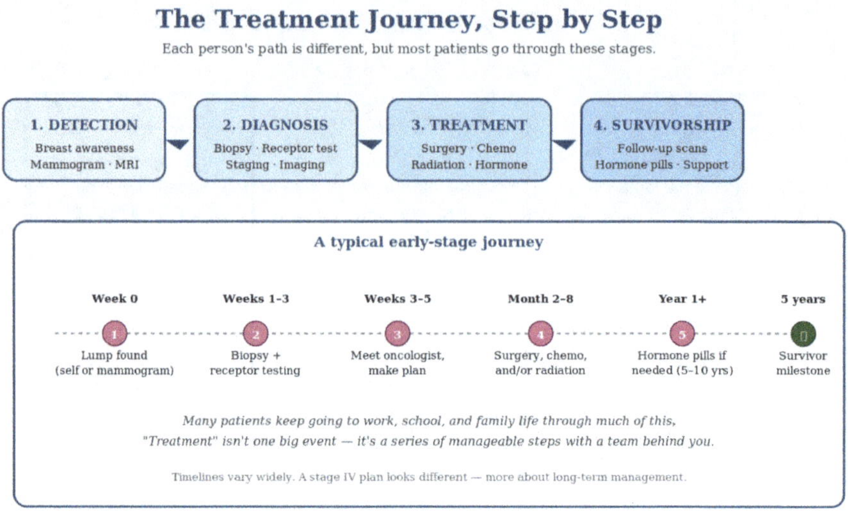

Figure 7.2 — The four phases of breast cancer care: Detection → Diagnosis → Treatment → Survivorship.

Surgery

Surgery is a common part of treatment for early-stage breast cancer, but it is not always the first step. Some patients receive chemotherapy, HER2-targeted therapy, immunotherapy, or other treatment before surgery to shrink the tumor or guide the plan. Two common breast operations are:

- **Lumpectomy:** The surgeon removes just the tumor and a small ring of healthy tissue around it (called a "margin"), keeping most of the breast. This is also called breast-conserving surgery. It is usually followed by radiation.
- **Mastectomy:** The surgeon removes the whole breast. Sometimes both are removed (a double, or bilateral, mastectomy), especially for women with BRCA mutations or a strong family history.

Surgeons will also usually check the lymph nodes under the arm. A sentinel node biopsy removes just one or two key nodes to test them; if those are clean, the rest can usually be left alone. If cancer is found in the sentinel node, the surgeon may remove more — called an axillary lymph node dissection. Removing many lymph nodes can cause a side effect called lymphedema, where the arm swells because lymph fluid can't drain. Modern care tries to minimize this with smarter, smaller surgeries.

Many women choose to have reconstructive surgery — rebuilding the breast with implants or with their own tissue (like skin and fat from the belly or back). Reconstruction can happen during the same surgery as the mastectomy, or months and years later. Some choose not to reconstruct at all and go "flat." There is no right answer. It is a personal decision.

Recovery varies widely depending on the operation, reconstruction, lymph-node surgery, overall health, and the work a person needs to return to. Some people recover quickly; others need several weeks or longer. The care team gives the safest timeline for lifting, driving, work, and exercise.

Radiation

Radiation uses high-energy rays (like super-powered X-rays) aimed exactly at where the tumor was. It kills any microscopic cancer cells that might have been left behind after surgery. Radiation is usually given as short appointments over 3 to 6 weeks, five days a week. Each session takes about 15–20 minutes — most of that is positioning. The actual radiation lasts a minute or two and you don't feel it.

Newer techniques like hypofractionated radiation give a higher dose over fewer days (sometimes just one week), with similar results and fewer side effects. Proton therapy, available at some major centers, uses particles instead of X-rays to spare nearby tissues — useful for people with breast cancer near the heart.

Radiation doesn't hurt during, but it can make the skin tired and red, like a sunburn. Tiredness builds toward the end of the course and lifts a few weeks after.

Chemotherapy

Chemo is strong medicine that travels through the whole body to kill cells that divide fast. That is great for killing cancer cells — and it is why hair (which divides fast) also falls out, why the lining of the mouth and stomach get sore, and why blood counts drop. Most side effects are temporary.

Modern chemo is given through an IV, usually over a few hours, every two or three weeks for several cycles. Many patients have a port placed under the skin so the IV doesn't need to be re-stuck each time. Anti-nausea medications today are far better than they were even ten years ago — most patients no longer spend days in bed sick.

Not everyone needs chemo. A big decision-maker is whether the cancer has or might have spread beyond the breast. For ER-positive cancers, doctors often run a special test called Oncotype DX or MammaPrint that looks at the genes inside the tumor and predicts whether chemo will help. This test has spared thousands of women from chemo they didn't need.

Hormone therapy

If a cancer is ER-positive or PR-positive, blocking hormones is a powerful weapon. Tamoxifen and aromatase inhibitors (like anastrozole, letrozole, exemestane) are pills that stop estrogen from feeding the cancer. Women often take them for 5 to 10 years after their main treatment to stop the cancer from coming back.

Hormone therapy can substantially lower the risk of recurrence for hormone-receptor-positive breast cancer. The benefit and duration depend on the individual cancer and patient. Side effects can include hot flashes, joint symptoms, mood changes, blood-clot risk with some drugs, and bone loss with aromatase inhibitors, so follow-up matters.

Targeted therapy

Targeted drugs are one of the biggest wins in modern cancer research. They are designed to lock onto a specific marker on cancer cells and ignore healthy cells. For HER2-positive cancer, drugs like trastuzumab (Herceptin), pertuzumab (Perjeta), and the newer trastuzumab deruxtecan (Enhertu) have transformed treatment — a disease that was once very scary is now much more beatable.

For some BRCA-related breast cancers, PARP inhibitors such as olaparib or talazoparib may be used. For many ER-positive/HER2-negative advanced cancers, CDK4/6 inhibitors such as ribociclib, abemaciclib, and others have improved disease control and, in several settings, overall survival. Which drug fits depends on the exact diagnosis and treatment line.

Immunotherapy

Immunotherapy is newer. Instead of attacking the cancer directly, these drugs train the person's own immune system to see and destroy cancer cells. Immunotherapy is especially promising for triple-negative breast cancer, which used to have almost no targeted options. Pembrolizumab (Keytruda) combined with chemo is now standard care for many patients with high-risk TNBC and has improved survival in real, measurable ways.

Clinical trials

A clinical trial is a research study that tests a new treatment in real patients. People sometimes think clinical trials are a "last resort." They are not. Many of the best treatments today became available because patients joined trials when they had other good options. Clinical trials are how cancer care moves forward.

If you or someone you love is diagnosed, it is fair to ask the oncologist: "Is there a clinical trial that might be right for me?" In the U.S., a free database at clinicaltrials.gov lists every active study. Many trials provide top-tier care and access to drugs that aren't yet on the market. Some specifically include Caribbean and Latin American patients to make sure new treatments work for our population.

Integrative and complementary care

"Integrative medicine" means using safe, evidence-backed things alongside standard treatments to help a person feel better during the fight. Research supports a few things in particular:

- Exercise. Appropriate activity during and after treatment can reduce fatigue, preserve strength and function, and improve quality of life. The care team can help adapt activity around surgery, blood counts, bone disease, neuropathy, or other limits.

- **Good nutrition.** A diet high in vegetables, fruit, whole grains, and lean protein supports the immune system. (See Chapter 8 for more.)
- **Mind-body practices.** Yoga, meditation, and prayer lower stress and help sleep. Chemotherapy is easier on a rested body.
- **Acupuncture.** Studies show it can reduce chemo-related nausea and joint pain from hormone therapy.
- Physical therapy and lymphedema care. These can help restore shoulder movement, manage swelling, reduce pain, and teach safe strategies after surgery. Massage may help some symptoms, but it is not a guaranteed way to prevent lymphedema.
- Support groups. Peer and family support can reduce isolation and improve coping and quality of life. They complement medical care; survival benefits are not guaranteed.
- **Counseling and therapy.** A diagnosis touches every part of life. Talking to a professional is a strength, not a weakness.

A careful note about "natural cures"

Some things sold as "natural cures" for cancer are dangerous, expensive, and pull people away from the treatments that actually work. High-dose supplements, strict juice-only diets, and "miracle" products have all

> *been linked to worse outcomes. If a product promises to cure cancer on its own — without a doctor — be very careful. Talk to the oncology team before starting anything new, even vitamins.*

What to ask the oncologist

It can be hard to think clearly in the doctor's office. Bring a notebook. Here are good questions to ask after a diagnosis:

- What type of breast cancer is this, and what stage?
- What are the receptors (ER, PR, HER2)?
- What is the proposed treatment plan, and why?
- Are there clinical trials I should consider?
- What are the most common side effects, and how do we manage them?
- How will treatment affect my work, family, fertility, or daily life?
- Should other family members be tested for genetic mutations?
- Who do I call when something doesn't feel right?
- Will I see the same team each time, or different doctors?
- Can my partner or family member sit in on appointments?

Chapter Eight.

Nutrition, Movement & Everyday Life

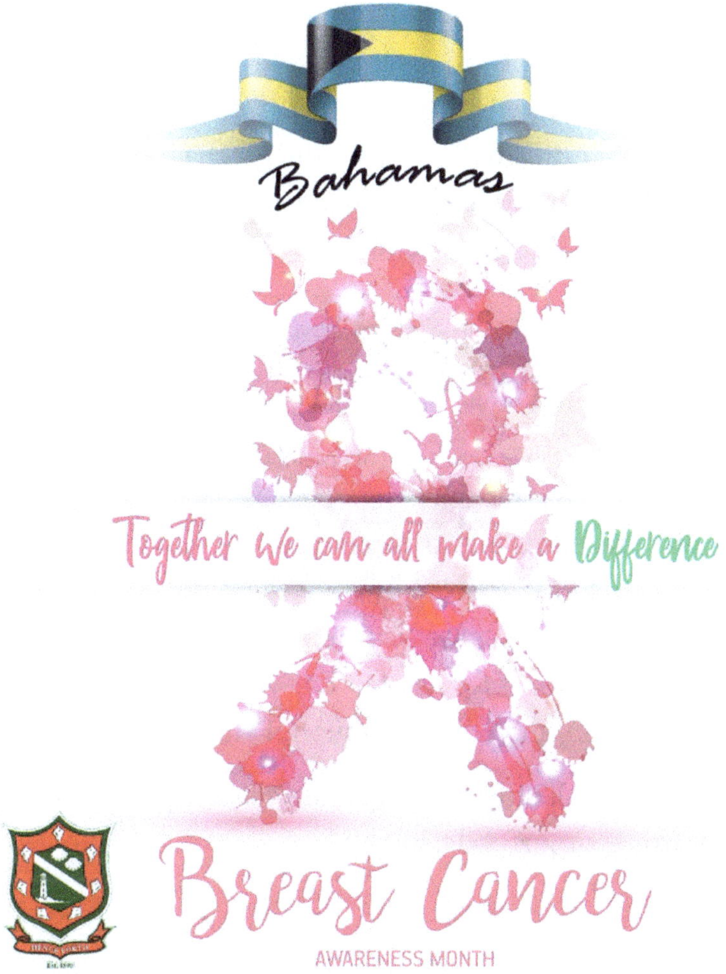

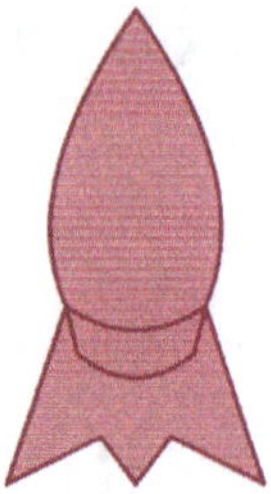

No food is a cure. No exercise is a guarantee. No sleep schedule makes anyone bulletproof. But lifestyle still matters: physical activity, alcohol intake, body weight after menopause, tobacco exposure, and overall diet can influence breast-cancer risk and general health. After a diagnosis, healthy habits can also support strength, recovery, and quality of life.

CUPCAKE CHECK – CHAPTER 8

No food or supplement cures breast cancer.
Regular activity, limited alcohol, healthy weight, and a balanced diet support overall risk reduction.
After diagnosis, nutrition and movement should be adapted to the treatment plan.

When I was researching this chapter, I expected to find a thousand "superfoods" that cure cancer. What I actually found was much simpler: the same boring, unsexy advice that doctors have been giving for fifty years. Eat more plants. Drink less alcohol. Move every day. Sleep enough. Don't smoke.

That advice is not flashy, but it is more trustworthy than a list of “cancer-fighting superfoods.”

Eating to protect your cupcakes

The most evidence-supported eating pattern is not a list of miracle foods. It is a mostly plant-forward pattern with vegetables, fruit, whole grains, beans, nuts, fish, and healthy fats, while limiting alcohol and heavily processed foods. A Mediterranean-style pattern fits that description, and Caribbean foods can fit it beautifully: callaloo, peas and beans, fish, avocado, citrus, papaya, mango, and whole grains.

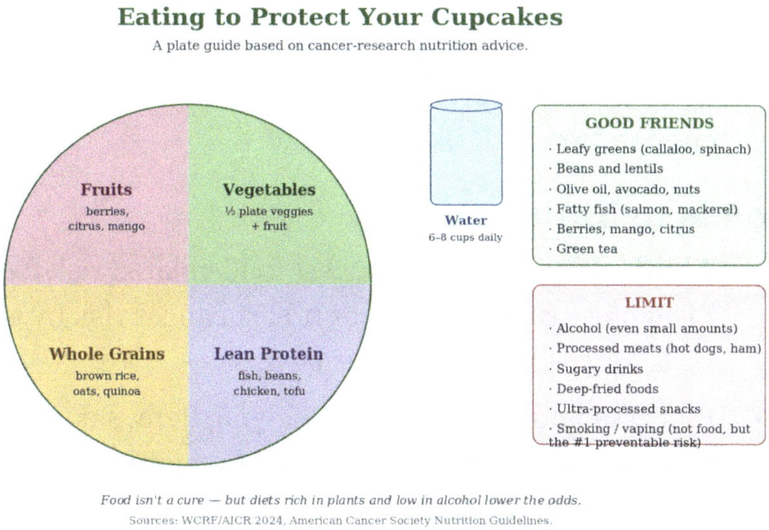

Figure 8.1 — A simple plate guide for cancer-aware eating.

Foods that the research consistently supports

- Leafy greens: callaloo, spinach, kale, collards. Nutrient-dense sources of folate, fiber, vitamins, and minerals.
- Cruciferous vegetables: broccoli, cauliflower, cabbage, brussels sprouts. Good sources of fiber and plant compounds; no single vegetable prevents cancer by itself.
- Beans and lentils: affordable fiber and plant protein that fit a healthy overall eating pattern.
- Berries and citrus: sources of vitamin C, fiber, and a variety of plant compounds.
- Fatty fish (salmon, mackerel, sardines): sources of protein and omega-3 fats that support cardiovascular health.

- **Whole grains:** brown rice, oats, quinoa, whole-wheat bread instead of white.
- **Nuts and seeds:** almonds, walnuts, flaxseed, chia.
- **Olive oil and avocado:** healthy fats that replace butter and palm oil.
- Green tea: reasonable as a beverage if you enjoy it, but evidence that it prevents breast cancer is not strong enough to treat it like medicine.

Foods to limit or avoid

- **Alcohol:** one of the strongest food-related risk factors. Even one drink a day raises breast cancer risk by about 7–10%. Less is better. None is best.
- Processed meats: hot dogs, bologna, ham, salami. Limit them as part of an overall cancer-prevention and heart-healthy eating pattern.
- Sugary drinks: soda and heavily sweetened drinks can add a lot of calories without much nutrition and can make healthy-weight goals harder.
- Ultra-processed snacks: many are high in sodium, refined starch, sugar, or saturated fat. They are better as occasional foods than the center of the diet.
- Deep-fried foods: an occasional fish fry can fit into real life. Frequency, portion size, and the rest of the eating pattern matter more than one meal.

Soy: a special note

A lot of women are told to avoid soy because they hear "estrogen" and panic. The research actually shows the opposite: moderate soy intake (tofu, edamame, soy milk, miso) is safe and may slightly reduce breast cancer risk and recurrence. The estrogens in soy are weak and behave differently than human estrogen. Avoid concentrated soy supplements or extracts, but normal soy foods are fine.

Move your body

Regular physical activity is one of the strongest modifiable habits linked with a lower breast-cancer risk. After a diagnosis, exercise can reduce fatigue, improve mood and function, and support overall health. The exact benefit varies from person to person, but movement is one of the most consistently useful tools we have.

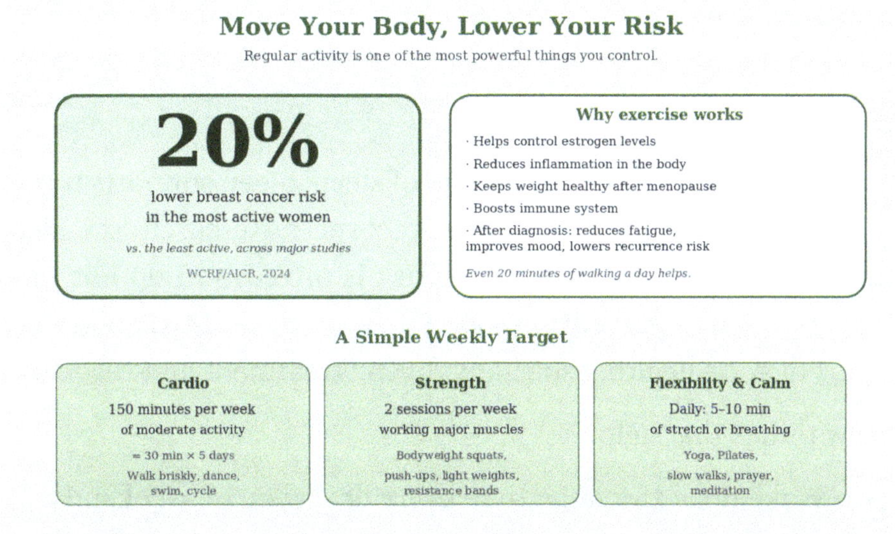

Figure 8.2 — A simple weekly target: 150 minutes of cardio, 2 strength sessions, and daily flexibility/calm.

You don't need a gym membership. Walking around your neighborhood counts. Dancing in your living room counts. Carrying groceries up the stairs counts. The American Cancer Society recommends:

- 150 minutes per week of moderate activity (or 75 minutes of vigorous), and
- Strength training 2 days per week.

Moderate means you can talk but not sing. Vigorous means you can only get out a few words at a time. Both are good.

After a diagnosis

Even during chemo and radiation, gentle exercise helps. Patients who walk regularly during treatment report less fatigue, better sleep, and better moods. Yoga and tai chi are especially well-studied for cancer patients. Always check with your team before starting anything new — but the answer is almost always "yes, please move."

Sleep

Most adults need about 7–9 hours of sleep. Sleep supports mood, energy, immune function, and recovery. Research on sleep duration itself and breast-cancer risk is mixed, so I do not want to oversell it as a prevention tool. I do want to say this: good sleep is part of good health, especially during treatment and recovery.

A few things that help:

- Wake up at the same time every day, even on weekends.
- Get morning sunlight within an hour of waking — it sets your body clock.
- No screens for the last 30 minutes before bed.
- Cool, dark, quiet room.
- No caffeine after lunch.

- A short wind-down ritual — reading, prayer, journaling, slow breathing.

Stress and mental health

Stress does not directly cause breast cancer. It can, however, disrupt sleep, worsen anxiety or depression, and make healthy routines harder to maintain. Caring for mental health is part of caring for physical health — especially during a diagnosis, treatment, or caregiving.

Things that genuinely help: regular movement, connection with people you love, time outside, creative work, prayer or meditation, and — when needed — therapy. There is no shame in asking for help. There is no badge for doing this alone.

Things to avoid

- **Smoking and vaping.** Smoking raises risk of breast cancer (especially in younger women) and many other cancers. Vaping is not safe — it is just less studied.
- **Tanning beds.** No proven link to breast cancer specifically, but tanning beds raise melanoma risk significantly.
- **Excessive supplements.** Multivitamins are fine. Mega-doses of single nutrients are not. More is not better.

> **The smallest change wins**
>
> *You don't have to overhaul your life this week. Pick one thing — one walk a day, one extra vegetable on your plate, one fewer drink — and stick with it for a month. Small habits beat big resolutions every time.*

Chapter Nine.

When Cancer Comes Home

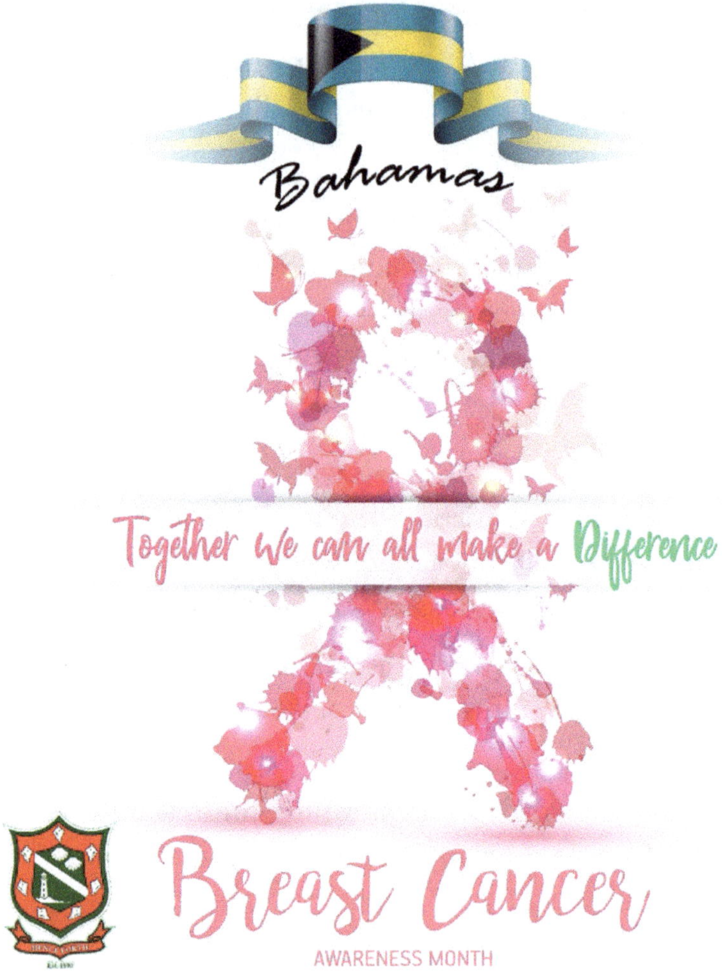

I want to talk to the people who don't usually get a chapter in cancer books: the kids and teens whose moms, aunts, grandmas, dads, or older siblings have been diagnosed. If that's you right now — or has been at some point — this chapter is for you.

> **CUPCAKE CHECK – CHAPTER 9**
>
> Young people deserve honest, age-appropriate information.
> You did not cause a loved one's cancer and you cannot cure it by being "perfect."
> Your own routine, school life, sleep, and support still matter.

When cancer comes home, the whole family enters a kind of fog. Adults are suddenly making appointments and decisions, sometimes whispering, sometimes crying, sometimes acting too cheerful. You may be told "everything is going to be fine," even when it doesn't feel fine. You may be told nothing at all, which is somehow worse. You may feel scared, angry, embarrassed, helpless, or completely numb. All of those reactions are normal.

Here's what I learned when my own family walked through it.

You are allowed to ask questions

Adults sometimes try to "protect" kids by hiding information. Most of the time, that backfires. Kids fill in the silence with their imagination, and their imagination is almost always worse than the truth.

You have the right to ask, in plain language:

- What kind of cancer is it?
- What is the treatment plan?
- Will she lose her hair?
- Will she be in the hospital?
- Is she going to die?

That last question is the hardest to ask. Ask it anyway. The honest answer — even if it's "we don't know yet" — is better than guessing in the dark.

You are not the cause and not the cure

Sometimes kids quietly believe that they did something to cause the cancer ("I was so mean to her last week"), or that they can cure it ("if I just behave perfectly, she'll get better"). Neither is true. Cancer is biology. It is not a punishment, and it is not a chore your family earned by something you did.

You also don't have to be the perfect kid through this. You're still allowed to argue with your sister, fail a test, have a bad day. Your job is to be a kid. Your job is not to fix this.

Things that might help your parent or relative

You may want to do something — anything — to help. Here are real ways teens and kids actually help:

- Bring her water. Patients in chemo get dehydrated; refilling the bottle is a small thing that means a lot.
- Be present. Sometimes she just needs you to sit beside her on the couch and watch a show.

- Let her see you. A patient stuck inside a "sick body" needs to remember she's also a mom, a sister, a friend.
- Take a chore off the list. Doing the dishes without being asked is a love language.
- Write her a note when treatment days are hard.
- Help younger siblings if you have them — they will follow your lead on how scared to be.

Take care of yourself, too

It can feel selfish to focus on yourself when someone you love is sick. It isn't. You are still growing, still going to school, still figuring out who you are. Those things matter.

Keep your routines as much as you can. Sleep at normal times. Eat real meals. See your friends. Move your body. Talk to a school counselor, a youth pastor, a coach, or a therapist if you need to. Many cancer hospitals have free programs for kids of patients — ask about CLIMB (Children's Lives Include Moments of Bravery) or similar local programs.

And cry when you need to. Crying is not weakness. It is the body's way of letting hard things move through.

Body image and feeling weird about your own body

When a parent has breast cancer, it can make you feel strange about your own body — especially if you are a teenage girl just starting to develop. You might catch yourself worrying about your own breasts more than usual. You might feel guilty for thinking about your body when your mom is sick. You might feel scared that you will get cancer too.

All of that is normal. Two things to remember:

- Your body is not your mom's body. Even if you carry a similar gene, you have your own life ahead of you, with screening, awareness, and (one day) decisions you can make for yourself. You are not doomed.
- Worrying about your body now is actually preparing you to take care of it later. Channel the worry into knowledge — that's what this whole book is for.

When the news is hard

Sometimes the news doesn't go the way the family hoped. Treatment doesn't work as planned. The cancer comes back. The conversations get more serious. If that happens, please remember:

- Bad news doesn't mean it's over. People live with stage IV breast cancer for years now, often many years.
- But if the worst does come, you are not alone. Hospice, palliative care, school counselors, faith communities, and grief therapists exist for a reason.
- It is okay to be both heartbroken and proud of your person at the same time.
- Carrying her story forward — telling people about her, about what she taught you — is one of the most powerful ways to keep her with you.

A few words for boys

Boys love their moms, sisters, aunts, and grandmas just as much as girls do. But sometimes boys are taught (often without anyone meaning to) that this isn't their topic — that breast cancer is "a girls' thing." It isn't.

You can sit through a chemo appointment. You can drive your mom to a check-up when you're old enough. You can read this book and pass it to your sister. You can ask your dad if anyone in your family has had cancer. You can — when the time comes — be the partner who reminds your wife to schedule her mammogram. You can be the dad who teaches your daughter that her body matters.

Quiet, steady men are some of the best caregivers in this story. Be one.

A note from Raquell

I started this book at thirteen, partly because I wanted other girls my age to feel less alone. If you are reading this in a hospital waiting room, on a couch next to your mom, or in your bedroom while the house is too quiet — I am thinking about you. You are not too young to understand what is happening, and you are not too young to help.

Chapter Ten.

Support, Family & Hope

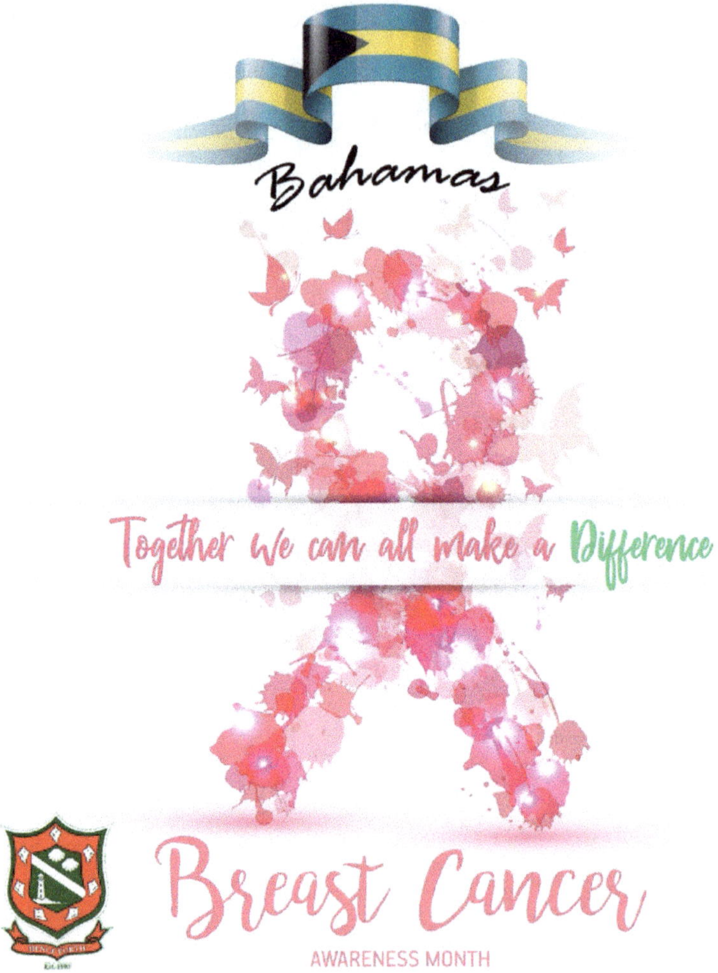

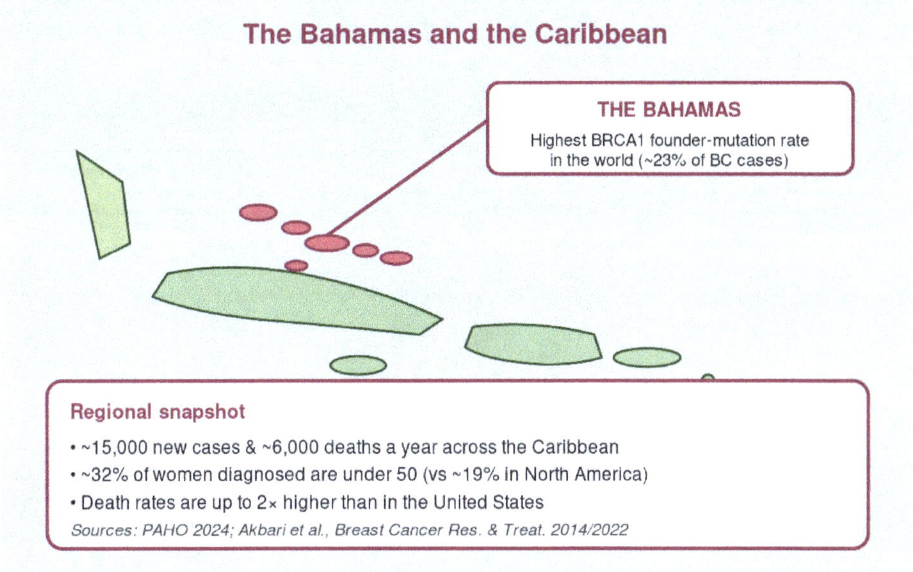

Figure 10.1 — Patients heal best when they are surrounded by people who show up.

A breast cancer diagnosis is not just one person's story. It belongs to a whole circle of people — the patient, her partner, her children, her parents, her siblings, her best friend, her pastor, her coworkers, the lady from down the street who drops off soup. Healing happens inside that circle. Without it, even the best medicine struggles.

This chapter is about what that circle looks like, how to be a part of one, and how to keep your own hope alive when the road gets long.

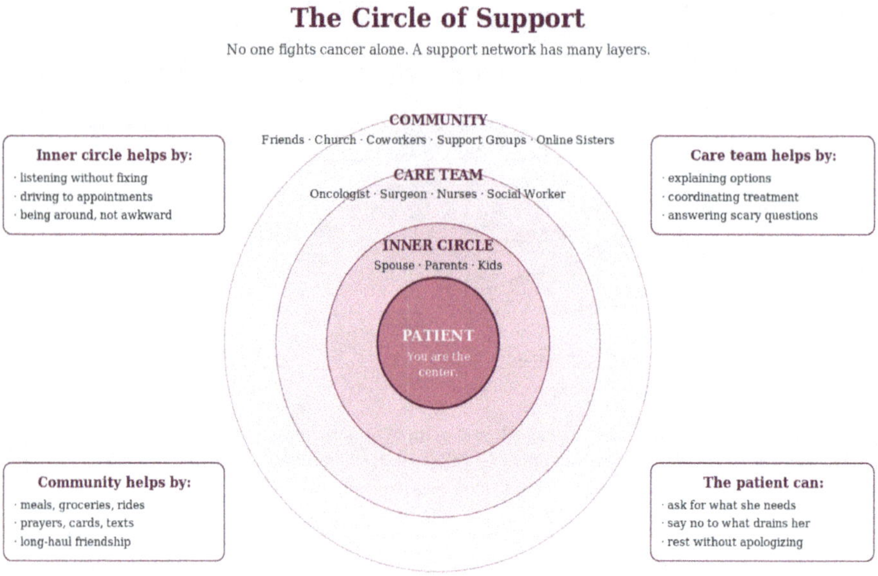

Figure 10.2 — The layered circle of support: from inner family out to community.

What survivors say they actually need

Researchers have asked thousands of breast cancer survivors what kind of help mattered most. The answers are surprisingly simple, and surprisingly easy for any of us to do:

- **Practical help.** Meals delivered, kids picked up from school, the dog walked, the laundry folded, a ride to the hospital. Small acts that take a giant weight off.
- **Specific offers, not "let me know if you need anything."** Try: "I'm bringing dinner Tuesday — chicken or fish?" or "I'm driving you to chemo Friday morning, I'll be at your house at 8."
- **Listening without fixing.** Sometimes the patient just needs to talk. You don't need to find the right words. "I'm here, and I'm not going anywhere" is enough.

- **Being treated like a person, not a diagnosis.** Talk about regular life. Movies. Gossip. The neighbor's wedding. Cancer is exhausting; normal life is medicine.
- **Long-term presence.** The first month after diagnosis is full of casseroles. Month six is quieter. Month twelve, even quieter. The friends who are still showing up at month twelve are the ones survivors remember forever.

How to talk to someone who has been diagnosed

A lot of people freeze. They don't know what to say, so they say nothing — and then later they wish they'd said something. Here are a few things that almost always land well:

> *"I'm so sorry you are going through this. I'm here. What can I do this week?"*

> *"I love you. That's it. I just wanted to say it out loud today."*

> *"I've been thinking about you. No need to write back."*

Things to avoid: "Everything happens for a reason." "My great-aunt had it and she didn't make it." "Have you tried apricot seeds?" "You're so brave." (Many survivors say "brave" feels like pressure to perform.) When in doubt, say less and listen more.

Caregiver burnout is real

If you are the partner, the daughter, the son, the parent — you are also going through this. Caregivers are at higher risk for depression, sleep problems, and physical illness during their loved one's treatment. You cannot pour from an empty cup.

- Trade off shifts with another family member if you can. No one person can be on duty 24/7 for a year.
- Keep going to your own doctor. Your own checkups don't pause because someone you love is sick.
- Find a caregiver support group. The Cancer Society of The Bahamas, Susan G. Komen, and CancerCare all run them, online and in person.
- Sleep is not optional. Eat real food. Move your body. These are not luxuries during a long fight — they are part of how you stay in it.
- Cry when you need to. Laugh when you can. Both are signs you're still here.

Faith, prayer, and finding meaning

For many families in The Bahamas and across the Caribbean, faith is the backbone of the cancer journey. Studies have found that patients who draw on a spiritual practice — whether that is Christian prayer, meditation, Rastafarian reflection, or another tradition — report lower anxiety and a stronger sense of purpose during treatment. Faith does not replace medicine. But for many, it carries the weight that medicine can't carry.

If your family prays, pray together. If your family doesn't, find your own quiet practice — a daily walk, journaling, music. The point is the same: leave a window open inside your own mind for hope to come through.

Survivorship: life after treatment

"Survivorship" is the word doctors use for the long stretch of life after active treatment ends. People expect this to feel like a finish line. It often doesn't. Survivors describe a strange mix of relief and fear, gratitude and grief. The body is healing but the mind is still catching up.

Most survivors will have follow-up visits every 3–6 months for the first few years, then once a year. Hormone-receptor-positive patients keep taking pills for years. Some live with low-grade side effects — joint stiffness, neuropathy in the hands or feet, lymphedema, "chemo brain" (a foggy memory and concentration problem) — that gradually improve over months and years.

Ten years after diagnosis, most early-stage breast cancer patients are alive and well. The world has been quietly rebuilt. New routines, new perspectives, sometimes new careers, new friendships forged in waiting rooms. As survivors say: cancer takes things from you, but it also gives you back a sharper sense of what matters.

Living with metastatic (Stage IV) breast cancer

A smaller group of women live with metastatic breast cancer — cancer that has spread beyond the breast and lymph nodes to other organs. Stage IV breast cancer is treatable but, with today's science, not curable for most patients. The goal becomes living with it, not beating it — like managing a serious chronic disease.

Thanks to new targeted drugs, immunotherapy, and CDK4/6 inhibitors, women with metastatic disease today are living longer than ever — often many years, sometimes decades, with active, full lives. Patients in the metastatic community describe a different kind of bravery: not "fighting until cured" but "living fully right now." Both kinds of bravery deserve respect.

If someone you love has metastatic breast cancer, the rules above still apply. Be present. Show up. Treat them like a person, not a prognosis. Help them live, not just survive.

Hope is a discipline

Hope is not just a feeling. Researchers who study cancer patients describe hope as a practice — something you do, on purpose, on the days you don't feel like it. You write down the small wins. You celebrate the milestones (last chemo, last radiation, first day back to work). You keep eyes on the next horizon — your daughter's graduation, your sister's wedding, the trip you promised yourself.

Hope is not naïve. It is honest. Hope sees the road clearly and chooses to keep walking. Hope is what every woman in this book has shown me — the patients, the survivors, my aunt, the women I will never meet whose stories changed how I see the world.

Takeaway

Healing takes more than medicine. It takes a circle of people who refuse to let anyone walk alone.

Be specific in your support. Be patient. Be present. Be there in month six, not just week one.

And remember: hope is a discipline. Practice it on purpose, especially on the hard days.

Chapter Eleven.

How You Can Help

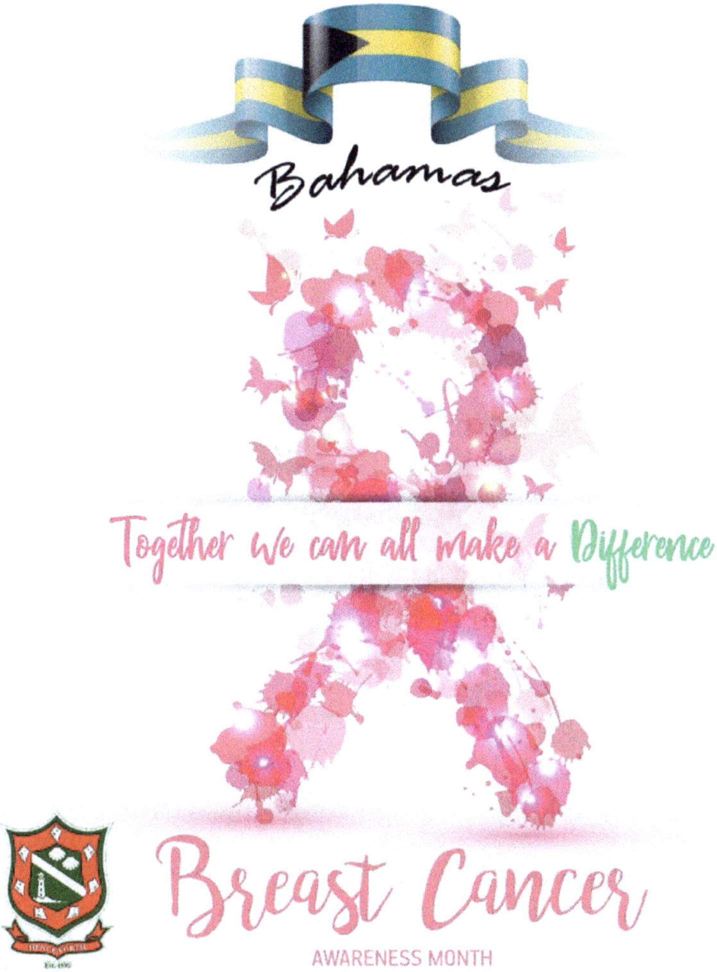

You finished a whole book about breast cancer. That already puts you ahead of most people. But knowledge sitting on a shelf doesn't save anyone. The next step is doing something with what you know.

CUPCAKE CHECK – CHAPTER 11

Pick one useful action and do it.
Use reliable sources and local organizations.
Advocacy can start in a classroom, family, church, workplace, or community group.

This chapter is a kind of menu. Pick one thing — even just one — and try it. Then come back and pick another.

If you are a student

- Talk to one woman in your life this week. Ask her if she has had a mammogram or done a self-exam recently. Tell her you read about it. You will be embarrassed for ten seconds. She will remember it for the rest of her life.
- Start a small awareness club at your school. October is Breast Cancer Awareness Month — ask permission to host a pink-shirt day, a bake sale, or a guest speaker.
- Volunteer with the Cancer Society of The Bahamas (or your local chapter). They always need help with packaging mammogram kits, running events, and visiting patients.
- Write. A poem, a song, a story, a TikTok. Art makes hard topics easier for other young people to absorb.
- Take a free CPR or first-aid class. Caregivers and patients deal with emergencies more often than most people. Knowing what to do matters.

If you are an adult

- Schedule your own screening — today. Mammograms get postponed for a million reasons. Make yours non-negotiable.
- Encourage three other women to do the same. Make a group text. Make a pact.
- Donate. Even a small amount, given monthly, funds research, free mammograms, and patient support. Susan G. Komen, the American Cancer Society, and Sister Sister Bahamas all accept recurring gifts.
- Drive a patient to a treatment appointment. Most cancer organizations have ride programs that need volunteers.
- Ask your employer to host an awareness session in October.
- Mentor a young person through a school health-club or scholarship program. The next generation of health workers, advocates, and researchers is looking for someone to follow.

If you are a teacher or school leader

- Add age-appropriate breast and reproductive health education to your science or health classes. Boys included — they will be partners and dads someday.
- Use this book as a discussion guide. The infographics make great classroom posters.
- Invite a survivor or oncologist to speak. Hearing from a real person turns information into something students remember.

- Support students who are dealing with a parent's diagnosis. Quiet check-ins. A flexible deadline. A note that says "I see you." It matters.

If you are a community leader, business owner, or church

- Sponsor a free mammogram day in your community.
- Make sure women in your organization who are 40+ have time off — without questions — to attend screenings.
- Distribute educational materials in waiting rooms, lobbies, and pews.
- Build a "meal train" or "ride train" system that activates whenever someone in the community is diagnosed. Most communities don't have one — until they do, and then they wonder how they ever did without it.

Advocacy in The Bahamas and the Caribbean

Some of the most important work in our region right now is happening at the policy level — pushing for better insurance coverage of mammograms, expanded BRCA genetic testing, and earlier screening for women at higher risk.

You can help by:

- Writing letters or emails to your Member of Parliament about cancer-screening access.
- Joining the Sister Sister Breast Cancer Support Group as a volunteer or junior advocate.

- Sharing real stories — your aunt's, your mom's, your neighbor's — when policy debates come up. Stories move people in ways that statistics cannot.
- Asking the Ministry of Health questions, in public, about how the country is investing in women's health.

A challenge

Pick one thing. Just one. Set a date next to it. Tell someone you're going to do it.

That is how this book stops being words on a page and starts being something real.

> **My promise to readers**
>
> *I am not finished with this work. I am studying so I can keep contributing to it as a young scientist. If you do something inspired by this book — anything, big or small — and want to share it with me, please write. Your story will keep me going on the days I need it.*

Conclusion: Protect Your Cupcakes

When I started writing this book in grade 8, I called it Protect Your Cupcakes because that's what girls my age called our breasts back then — sweet, ours, and worth taking care of. I didn't know then how much that little title would carry.

Now, six years later, "protect your cupcakes" means something bigger to me. It means: protect yourself. Protect your mom, your sister, your aunt, your grandma. Protect the women who raised you and the women you might raise one day. Protect the part of yourself that is brave enough to ask hard questions, and the part of yourself that is soft enough to keep loving people through hard answers.

What this book has been about

We started by understanding how the breast works and what cancer actually is. We went into the different types — DCIS, IDC, ILC, the rare ones — and the receptor subtypes that drive what kind of treatment a person gets. We talked about stages, warning signs, what to do at the doctor's office, and how genes like BRCA1 and BRCA2 — and especially the founder mutation we now know is more common in Bahamian women — change the conversation completely.

We talked about screening, and why early detection saves lives. We took the time, in our own chapter, to look at what is happening here in The Bahamas and across the Caribbean — and why the women in our region are diagnosed younger and with more aggressive disease than women in many other parts of the world.

We walked through every major treatment, including the newer ones (targeted drugs, immunotherapy, clinical trials) that didn't exist when our grandmothers were young. We added a whole chapter on lifestyle — what to eat, how to move, how to sleep, how to handle stress — because it turns out the day-to-day matters more than people used to think.

We talked to young people, especially daughters and sons watching a parent go through cancer. We talked about caregivers, about hope as a discipline, and about all the ways an ordinary person can take action.

What I hope you walk away with

- Breast cancer is common, but it is not undefeatable. Caught early, it is one of the most survivable cancers we know.
- Knowing your body is the most powerful tool you have. Self-awareness, self-exams, screening — these are all free or close to it, and they save lives.
- Genes matter. If breast or ovarian cancer runs in your family, ask about BRCA testing. If you are Bahamian, that conversation might apply to you even when you think it doesn't.
- You don't have to be a doctor to make a difference. You just have to be informed and willing to speak up.
- Hope is not a feeling we wait for. It is something we choose, and re-choose, every single day.

A final word

Six years ago I was thirteen, standing on a stage at Queens College talking about a disease I barely understood. I thought I knew what brave looked like back then. I didn't. I learned what brave looked like by watching my aunt Lorna, by watching the women at the Cancer Society, by reading the stories of survivors I will never meet. I learned what brave looked like by losing my grandfather to cancer and choosing to study oncology because of him, not in spite of him.

Brave is not the absence of fear. Brave is reading this book even though parts of it scared you. Brave is making the appointment. Brave is having the conversation with your mom or your daughter. Brave is sitting next to someone in a waiting room.

Brave is also small. Brave is taking one minute, in the shower, to know your own body. Brave is one phone call. Brave is one honest sentence to someone you love.

I will keep writing, keep studying, keep showing up. I hope you will too.

Protect your cupcakes. Protect each other. The next chapter belongs to you.

— Raquell

Nassau, The Bahamas · 2026

Glossary

Plain-language definitions of words used in this book. If you see a word here you don't recognize, this is the place to look it up.

Adjuvant therapy. Treatment given after surgery (chemo, hormone therapy, radiation, targeted therapy) to lower the chance the cancer comes back.

Aromatase inhibitor. A class of pills (anastrozole, letrozole, exemestane) that lower estrogen in the body. Used in postmenopausal women with HR-positive cancer.

Axillary lymph node dissection. Surgery to remove most of the lymph nodes in the armpit. Done if cancer has clearly spread to several nodes.

Benign. Not cancer. A benign lump is not dangerous, even if it has to be removed.

Biopsy. Removing a small sample of tissue or cells to look at under a microscope. The only way to know for sure if a lump is cancer.

BRCA1 / BRCA2. Genes that, when mutated, sharply raise the risk of breast and ovarian cancer. A specific BRCA1 mutation is more common in Bahamian women than in almost any other group.

Carcinoma. Cancer that starts in the lining of organs. Most breast cancers are carcinomas (ductal or lobular).

CDK4/6 inhibitor. Newer pills (palbociclib, ribociclib, abemaciclib) used for HR-positive metastatic breast cancer. Major life-extending breakthrough.

Chemotherapy ("chemo"). Strong medicine that kills fast-dividing cells throughout the body. Used to kill cancer cells that have spread or might spread.

Clinical trial. A research study that tests new treatments. Often gives access to drugs years before they become widely available.

CT scan. A detailed X-ray that shows cross-sections of the body. Used to look for spread.

DCIS (Ductal Carcinoma In Situ). Stage 0 cancer. Abnormal cells inside the milk duct that haven't spread. Highly curable.

Estrogen receptor (ER). A protein on some cancer cells that lets estrogen feed the cancer. ER-positive cancers can be treated with hormone therapy.

Fibroadenoma. A common, harmless lump made of breast tissue. Not cancer.

Genetic counseling. Meeting with a specialist who explains the risks and benefits of genetic testing and helps interpret results.

Grade. How abnormal the cancer cells look (1 = looks close to normal; 3 = looks very abnormal and aggressive).

HER2 (Human Epidermal Growth Factor Receptor 2). A protein on some cancer cells. HER2-positive cancers grow fast but respond to targeted drugs like Herceptin.

Hormone receptor (HR). Either ER or PR. HR-positive cancers grow on hormones; treated with hormone-blocking pills.

Hormone therapy. Pills like tamoxifen and aromatase inhibitors that block hormones from feeding HR-positive cancers.

IDC (Invasive Ductal Carcinoma). The most common kind of breast cancer (~70–80%). Cancer that started in a duct and spread into nearby tissue.

ILC (Invasive Lobular Carcinoma). About 10–15% of cases. Starts in the lobules and can be harder to feel as a lump.

Immunotherapy. Drugs that train the body's own immune system to attack cancer. Used in some triple-negative cases.

Inflammatory breast cancer (IBC). A rare, fast-moving kind that makes the breast look red and swollen. Needs urgent care.

Invasive cancer. Cancer that has broken out of the duct or lobule and started growing into nearby breast tissue.

Ki-67. A test that measures how fast a cancer is dividing. Higher = faster growing.

LCIS (Lobular Carcinoma In Situ). Not technically cancer, but a warning sign that risk is higher.

Lumpectomy. Surgery that removes only the tumor and a margin of healthy tissue, keeping most of the breast.

Lymph node. Small bean-shaped filters of the immune system. Doctors check the ones under the arm because cancer often spreads to them first.

Lymphedema. Swelling (often of the arm) caused by removed or damaged lymph nodes. Managed with massage, exercise, and compression sleeves.

Malignant. Cancerous. The opposite of benign.

Mammogram. A low-dose X-ray of the breast used to find cancer early.

Mastectomy. Surgery that removes the entire breast.

Metastasis (Stage IV). When cancer has spread to other organs (bones, lungs, liver, brain). Treatable, often for years, but not usually curable.

MRI. A detailed scan using magnets. Used in addition to mammograms for very dense breasts or high-risk patients.

Neoadjuvant therapy. Treatment (often chemo) given before surgery to shrink the tumor.

Oncologist. A doctor who specializes in cancer.

Oncotype DX / MammaPrint. Tests that look at the genes inside a tumor to predict whether chemo will help.

Palliative care. Care focused on relieving symptoms and improving quality of life. Can happen alongside curative treatment, not just at the end.

PARP inhibitor. A class of drugs (olaparib, talazoparib) used for BRCA-related cancers.

Pathology. The study of tissue under a microscope. The pathology report tells the rest of the team what kind of cancer this is.

Port (port-a-cath). A small device placed under the skin that lets nurses give chemo without sticking the arm every time.

Progesterone receptor (PR). Like ER, a protein that lets the hormone progesterone fuel a cancer. PR-positive cancers respond to hormone therapy.

Radiation therapy. High-energy beams that kill any cancer cells left after surgery.

Reconstruction. Surgery to rebuild the breast after a mastectomy, using implants or the patient's own tissue.

Recurrence. When cancer comes back after treatment.

Sentinel node biopsy. Removing only the first one or two lymph nodes the cancer would spread to and testing them.

Stage. How far the cancer has spread (Stage 0–IV). Lower stage = better prognosis.

Survivorship. Life after active treatment ends. Includes follow-up care, side-effect management, and emotional recovery.

Targeted therapy. Drugs that lock onto a specific marker on cancer cells (like HER2 or BRCA) and ignore healthy cells.

Triple-negative breast cancer (TNBC). Cancer that is ER-, PR-, and HER2-negative. More common in Black women, young women, and women with BRCA1.

Tumor. A lump made of abnormal cells. Tumors can be benign or malignant.

Ultrasound. Imaging that uses sound waves. Used to look at lumps, especially in younger women with dense breasts.

A Few Words in Spanish & Haitian Creole

The Caribbean is not one language. If English isn't the easiest language for someone you love, these few words may help start the conversation.

- **Breast.** Spanish: Seno · Haitian Creole: Tete
- **Lump.** Spanish: Bulto · Haitian Creole: Boul
- **Cancer.** Spanish: Cáncer · Haitian Creole: Kansè
- **Doctor.** Spanish: Médico · Haitian Creole: Doktè
- **Mammogram.** Spanish: Mamografía · Haitian Creole: Mamogram
- **Family history.** Spanish: Antecedentes familiares · Haitian Creole: Istwa medikal fanmi
- **Early detection.** Spanish: Detección temprana · Haitian Creole: Detekte bonè
- **Support group.** Spanish: Grupo de apoyo · Haitian Creole: Gwoup sipò

These are offered as a starting point, not a certified translation — please have a fluent speaker check them before they go to print.

Resources & Hotlines

If you or someone you love needs help, information, or just someone to talk to, the following organizations are good places to start. (Information was current as of early 2026 — always confirm the latest number or website.)

In The Bahamas

- Cancer Society of The Bahamas. Cancer education, patient/family support, Caring Centre accommodations, Family Island programs, and other services. (242) 323-4441 / 323-4482 · cancersocietybahamas.org
- Sister Sister Breast Cancer Support Group. Bahamian peer support, screening and awareness programs, and community advocacy. Centreville Medical Center, 68 Collins Avenue, Nassau · (242) 326-1929 · sistersisterbahamas.com
- Ask about cost before you skip a screening. Cost is one of the reasons care gets delayed in The Bahamas. The Fox Foundation's free breast-exam days during Breast Cancer Awareness Month and the Cancer Society of The Bahamas both exist because of this. If a mammogram, biopsy, or follow-up feels unaffordable, ask the clinic or the Cancer Society directly about payment plans, sliding-scale fees, or a referral to a free program before deciding to wait.
- Ask local cancer organizations and clinics about current Breast Cancer Awareness Month screening events. Programs can change from year to year, so confirm directly before relying on an event or location.

- Princess Margaret Hospital — Oncology Services. Shirley Street, Nassau. Main switchboard: (242) 322-2861. Confirm clinic extensions and appointment instructions with the hospital.
- The Bahamas Crisis Centre. 24-hour crisis hotline: (242) 328-0922; WhatsApp textline: (242) 565-9633. Its core work focuses on violence/abuse crisis support and counseling; for immediate danger in The Bahamas call 919.

Across the Caribbean

- **Jamaica Cancer Society.** jamaicacancersociety.org · (876) 927-4265.
- **Trinidad & Tobago Cancer Society.** cancer.tt · (868) 226-4267.
- **Barbados Cancer Society.** cancersociety.bb
- **Pan American Health Organization (PAHO).** Region-wide statistics, prevention guidelines, and country reports. paho.org

International

- **American Cancer Society.** 24/7 helpline: 1-800-227-2345 · cancer.org
- **Susan G. Komen.** Helpline: 1-877-465-6636 · komen.org
- **National Cancer Institute (USA).** cancer.gov · 1-800-422-6237
- **CancerCare.** Free counseling, support groups, and resources. 1-800-813-4673 · cancercare.org
- **Living Beyond Breast Cancer.** lbbc.org
- **Metavivor (for metastatic patients).** metavivor.org

- **BRCA Strong (community for previvors and BRCA carriers).** brcastrong.org
- **ClinicalTrials.gov.** Searchable database of every active clinical trial in the U.S. clinicaltrials.gov

If you are struggling emotionally

A cancer diagnosis (your own or someone you love's) can bring up depression, anxiety, or thoughts of giving up. You are not alone, and help is available.

- The Bahamas Crisis Centre: (242) 328-0922; WhatsApp (242) 565-9633 (crisis support, especially violence/abuse-related).
- **In the U.S., call or text 988** (Suicide & Crisis Lifeline).
- **CancerCare counseling.** 1-800-813-4673 (free counselors who specialize in cancer).

If you or someone near you is in immediate danger, please go to the nearest emergency room or call your local emergency number right away.

Quick Reference — Take This With You

Photograph this page, tear it out, or copy it onto an index card. It's everything in this book you need in a hurry.

The 5-Step Awareness Check

- **Step 1 — Look.** Mirror, hands on hips, shoulders straight. Look for changes in size, shape, or color.
- **Step 2 — Look again.** Same check, arms raised overhead — this pulls tissue tighter and makes changes easier to spot.
- **Step 3 — Check the nipple.** Watch for a new inversion, rash, or discharge that isn't milk.
- **Step 4 — Feel.** Lying down, small overlapping circles, collarbone to belly and chest to armpit, light/medium/firm pressure.
- **Step 5 — Repeat in the shower.** Wet, soapy skin makes changes easier to notice.

Warning Signs — See a Doctor If You Notice

- A new lump, especially one that's hard, uneven, or doesn't move
- Skin dimpling, like an orange peel
- A nipple that suddenly turns inward
- Fluid from the nipple that isn't breast milk, especially with blood in it

- Redness, rash, or warmth that won't heal
- Swelling or a change in shape on one side
- A lump in the armpit
- Pain in one spot that won't go away
- Anything that "doesn't feel right" — trust that instinct

Screening at a Glance (Average Risk)

- **ACS.** Ages 40–44: yearly mammogram is a personal choice
- **ACS.** Ages 45–54: yearly mammogram
- **ACS.** Age 55+: every 2 years, or continue yearly
- **USPSTF.** Ages 40–74: mammogram every 2 years
- Higher risk (BRCA, strong family history, prior chest radiation): ask about starting earlier and adding MRI

Numbers to Keep

- **Cancer Society of The Bahamas** — (242) 323-4441 / 323-4482
- **Sister Sister Breast Cancer Support Group** — (242) 326-1929
- **Princess Margaret Hospital, Oncology** — (242) 322-2861
- **The Bahamas Crisis Centre** — (242) 328-0922 · WhatsApp (242) 565-9633
- **American Cancer Society** — 1-800-227-2345, or 988 for the Suicide & Crisis Lifeline in the U.S.

One Sentence to Remember

A new change that lasts more than a couple of weeks is a reason to see a doctor — not someday. Soon.

Works Cited

This edition was updated against the following current guidance and source material, listed in MLA style. Medical recommendations change; readers should verify the latest version when making health decisions.

Akbari, M. R., et al. "The Spectrum of BRCA1 and BRCA2 Mutations in Breast Cancer Patients in the Bahamas." *Clinical Genetics*, vol. 85, no. 1, 2014, pp. 64-67, doi:10.1111/cge.12132.

American Cancer Society. "Breast Cancer Screening Guidelines and Recommendations for Early Detection." *American Cancer Society*, cancer.org.

---. *Cancer Facts & Figures 2026*. American Cancer Society, 2026.

---. "Key Statistics for Breast Cancer." *American Cancer Society*, 24 June 2026, cancer.org.

---. "Survival Rates for Breast Cancer." *American Cancer Society*, 23 July 2026, cancer.org.

Donenberg, T., et al. "A High Prevalence of BRCA1 Mutations among Breast Cancer Patients from the Bahamas." *Breast*

Cancer Research and Treatment, vol. 125, no. 2, 2011, pp. 591-96, doi:10.1007/s10549-010-1156-9.

International Agency for Research on Cancer. *Bahamas Country Report 2023: Cancers Amenable to Screening – Capacity and Response*. CanScreen5, IARC, 2023.

Narod, S. A., et al. "Follow-up of Bahamian Women with a BRCA1 or BRCA2 Mutation." *Molecular Genetics & Genomic Medicine*, vol. 6, no. 2, 2018, pp. 301-04.

National Cancer Institute. "BRCA Gene Changes: Cancer Risk and Genetic Testing." *National Cancer Institute*, cancer.gov.

---. "BRCA1 and BRCA2: Cancer Risks and Management (PDQ)." *National Cancer Institute*, Health Professional Version, cancer.gov.

---. "Causes and Risk Factors: Breast Cancer." *National Cancer Institute*, 2 Dec. 2025, cancer.gov.

Pan American Health Organization. *The Bahamas: Country Profile, Health in the Americas*. PAHO, 2024.

---, and World Health Organization. *Comprehensive Cancer Control Assessment in the Bahamas*. PAHO/WHO, 29 Apr. 2026.

Stuart, Raquell. *Protect Your Cupcakes: Understanding & Fighting Breast Cancer*. Original manuscript ed., 2020.

Trottier, M., et al. "Prevalence of Founder Mutations in the BRCA1 and BRCA2 Genes among Unaffected Women from the Bahamas." *Clinical Genetics*, vol. 89, no. 3, 2016, pp. 328-31, doi:10.1111/cge.12602.

United States, Preventive Services Task Force. "Breast Cancer: Screening." *Final Recommendation Statement*, 2024.

World Health Organization. "Global Breast Cancer Initiative." *World Health Organization*, who.int.

About the Author

Raquell Stuart

Raquell Stuart is a young Bahamian writer, advocate, and aspiring oncologist. She began writing Protect Your Cupcakes at the age of thirteen, during her year as Student of the Year at Queens College in Nassau. Her platform — breast cancer awareness — took her from her own classroom to the national stage, where she was named First Runner-Up for National Student of the Year of The Bahamas.

Throughout her platform, Raquell partnered with the Cancer Society of The Bahamas, raised funds for women affected by breast cancer, and traveled across the country to speak about prevention, screening, and survivorship. Her drive to study cancer was deepened by family loss — her grandfather, Clyde Ifill, passed away from pancreatic cancer — and by walking through her aunt's diagnosis and recovery alongside the rest of her family.

Raquell is currently pursuing her education with a focus on the medical sciences and plans to study oncology in the years ahead. Her goal is to one day combine clinical care with research that improves cancer outcomes for Caribbean women — particularly through better access to genetic testing, earlier screening, and culturally informed patient education.

When she is not studying or writing, Raquell enjoys reading, mentoring younger students, spending time with her family, and continuing the work that gave this book its name. She lives in Nassau, The Bahamas.

— —

Expanded Edition Editor & Project Lead

Cassius Stuart is Raquell Stuart's father and served as the expanded-edition editor and project lead for the 2026 revival of Protect Your Cupcakes. His role was to help shape the expanded structure, coordinate the editorial rebuild, strengthen sourcing, preserve Raquell's original voice, and bring the project back to publication six years after the first edition. Raquell Stuart remains the sole author of the book.

— —

To contact the author for school visits, speaking engagements, or community events, please write to the publisher.

THE END

— but really, the beginning. —

www.ingramcontent.com/pod-product-compliance
Lightning Source LLC
LaVergne TN
LVHW050824061126
851857LV00012B/962